It's easy to get lost in the cancer world

Let NCCN Guidelines for Patients® be your guide

- ✓ Step-by-step guides to the cancer care options likely to have the best results
- ✓ Based on treatment guidelines used by health care providers worldwide
- ✓ Designed to help you discuss cancer treatment with your doctors

About

NCCN Guidelines for Patients® are developed by the National Comprehensive Cancer Network® (NCCN®)

NCCN

- An alliance of leading cancer centers across the United States devoted to patient care, research, and education

Cancer centers that are part of NCCN:
NCCN.org/cancercenters

NCCN Clinical Practice Guidelines in Oncology (NCCN Guidelines®)

- Developed by doctors from NCCN cancer centers using the latest research and years of experience
- For providers of cancer care all over the world
- Expert recommendations for cancer screening, diagnosis, and treatment

Free online at
NCCN.org/guidelines

NCCN Guidelines for Patients

- Present information from the NCCN Guidelines in an easy-to-learn format
- For people with cancer and those who support them
- Explain the cancer care options likely to have the best results

Free online at
NCCN.org/patientguidelines

and supported by funding from NCCN Foundation®

These NCCN Guidelines for Patients are based on the NCCN Guidelines® for Survivorship (Version 2.2020, July 14, 2020).

NCCN Foundation seeks to support the millions of patients and their families affected by a cancer diagnosis by funding and distributing NCCN Guidelines for Patients. NCCN Foundation is also committed to advancing cancer treatment by funding the nation's promising doctors at the center of innovation in cancer research. For more details and the full library of patient and caregiver resources, visit NCCN.org/patients.

National Comprehensive Cancer Network (NCCN) / NCCN Foundation
3025 Chemical Road, Suite 100
Plymouth Meeting, PA 19462
215.690.0300

Sponsored by

gooddays

Good Days is proud to support this educational resource for patients and their families and offers unwavering commitment to those who struggle with chronic disease, cancer, and other life-altering conditions. mygooddays.org

Endorsed by

American Lung Association

The American Lung Association strongly supports efforts to help ensure all patients facing lung cancer get the highest standard of treatment and care. Helping patients understand treatment guidelines is one important step in empowering them to get the care they want and need. That is why we are pleased to endorse NCCN's efforts to provide accessible treatment guidelines and information to patients through the NCCN Guidelines for Patients. lung.org

Be The Match®

National Marrow Donor Program® (NMDP)/Be The Match® is the global leader in providing a possible cure to patients with life-threatening blood and marrow cancers, as well as other diseases. Our Be The Match Patient Support Center provides support, information, and resources for patients, caregivers, and families. BeTheMatch.org/one-on-one

Cancer Hope Network

As an organization committed to providing peer mentorship and ensuring that no one faces cancer alone, Cancer Hope Network is proud to endorse the informative, straightforward NCCN Patient Guidelines. These guidelines are a valuable tool for patients, caregivers and survivors, empowering them to live the best version of their lives while facing cancer. cancerhopenetwork.org

Save Your Skin Foundation

Save Your Skin Foundation (SYSF) is a Canadian patient-led not-for-profit group dedicated to the fight against non-melanoma skin cancers, melanoma and ocular melanoma. By using and sharing the valuable and thorough NCCN Guidelines, SYSF is confident in their provision of solid patient support with accurate and current information on these cancers and related topics such as skin cancer treatment with immunotherapy. saveyourskin.ca

The Leukemia & Lymphoma Society

The Leukemia & Lymphoma Society (LLS) is dedicated to developing better outcomes for blood cancer patients and their families through research, education, support and advocacy and is happy to have this comprehensive resource available to patients. lls.org/informationspecialists

With generous support from

Gena and Dan Cook
Crystal Denlinger, MD
- **in honor of Edgar and Cynthia Denlinger**
- **in honor of Joan McClure**

Kristina Gregory
Melissa Hudson, MD
Wui-Jin Koh, MD
- **in honor of Judith Anne Hanada Koh**

Terry Langbaum
Javid Moslehi, MD
Lindsay Peterson, MD
William Piri

To make a gift or learn more, please visit NCCNFoundation.org/donate or e-mail PatientGuidelines@nccn.org.

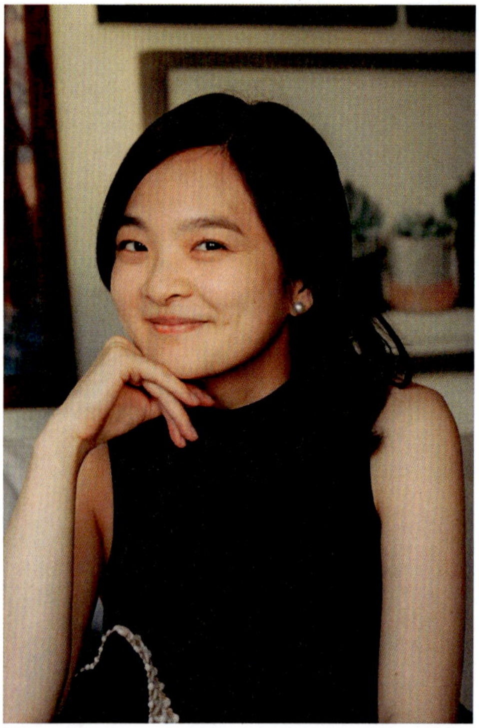
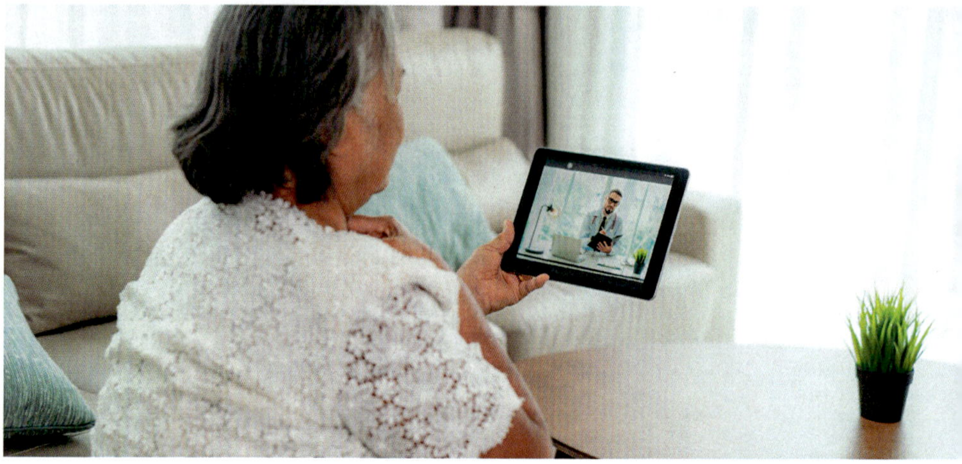
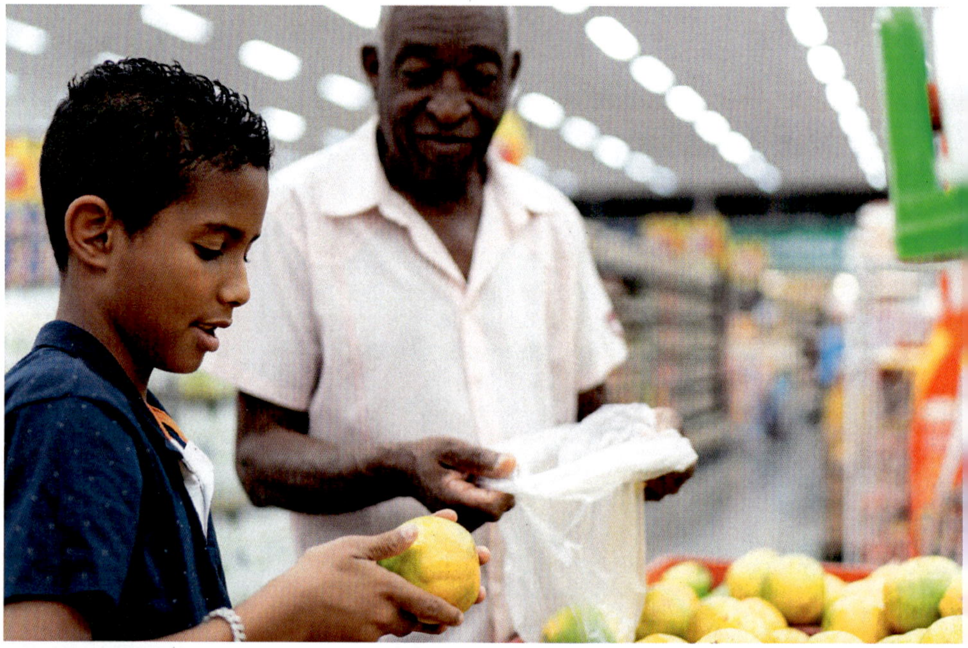
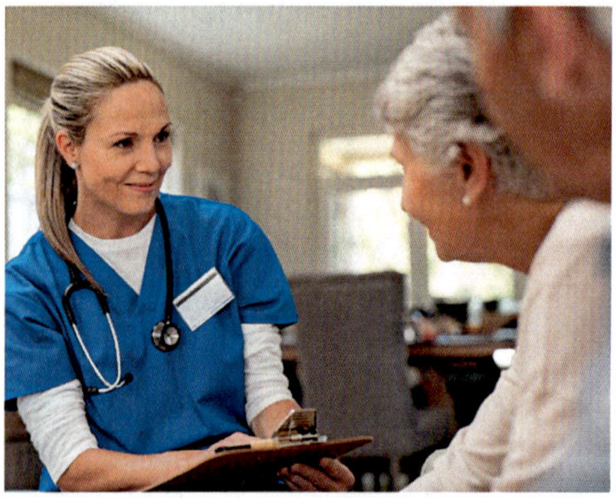
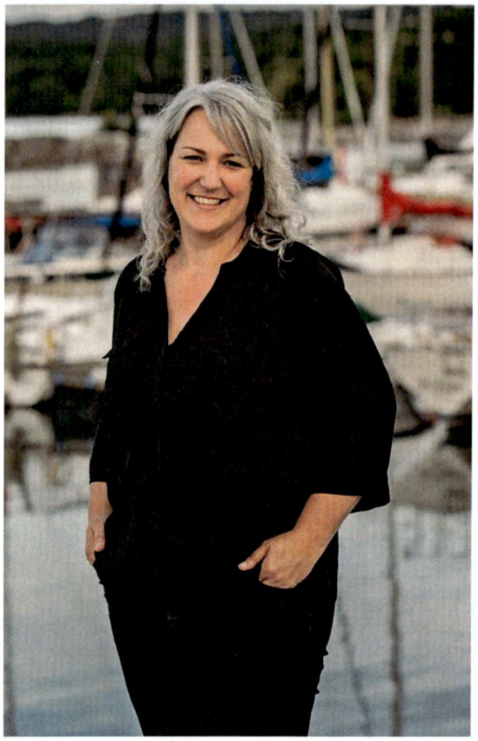
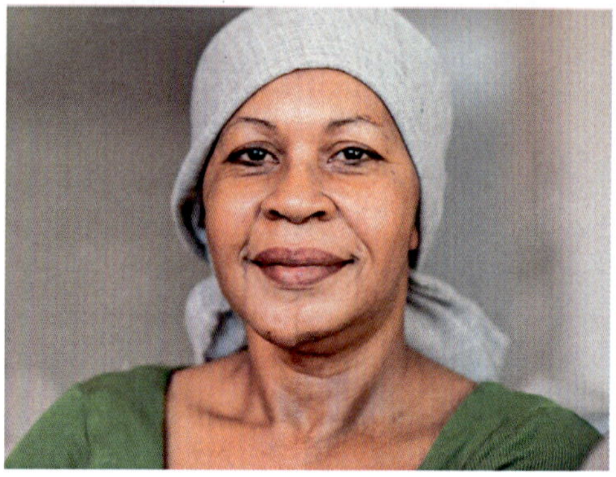
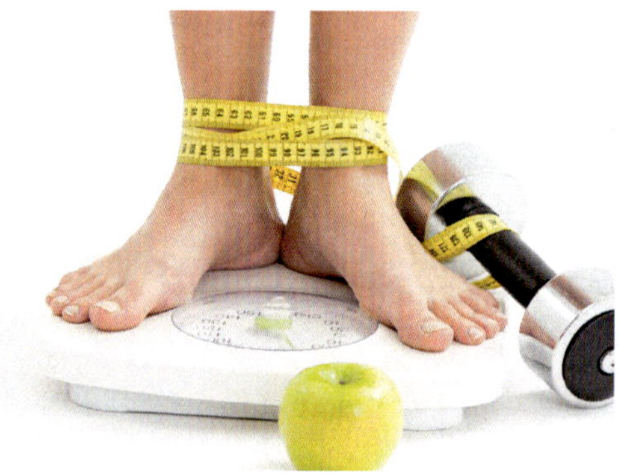
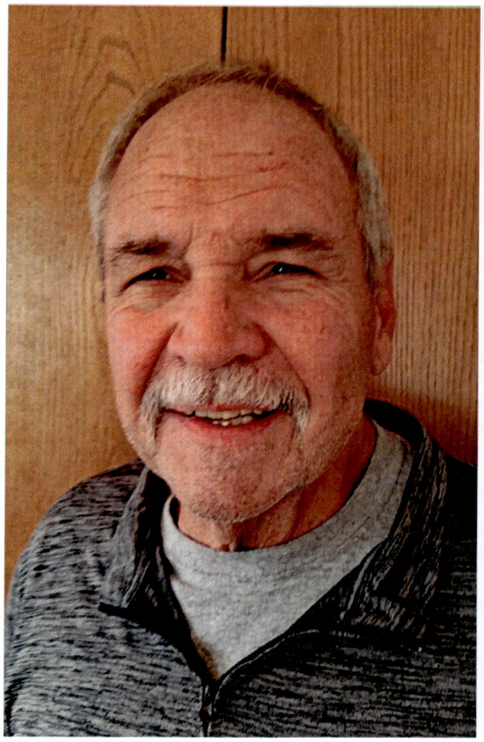

Contents

6 Survivorship

12 Physical activity

20 Food and supplements

29 Weight and metabolism

35 Preventing infections

41 Resources

47 Words to know

49 NCCN Contributors

50 NCCN Cancer Centers

51 Index

1 Survivorship

7 Cancer survivors

7 Survivorship care

9 Survivorship guidelines

10 Healthy living

11 Review

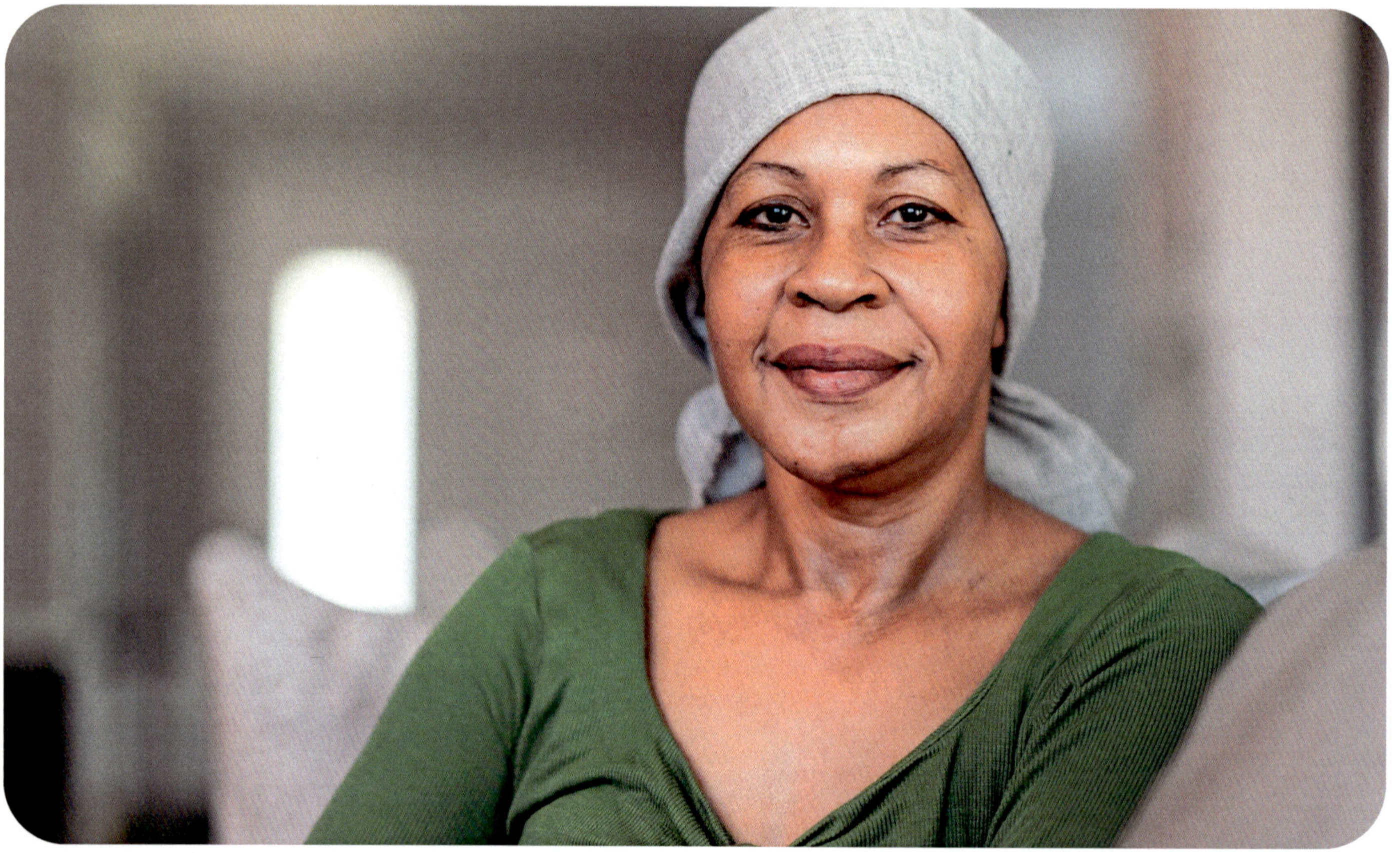

People with cancer are living longer than they did in the past. They are surviving, and their needs have changed. Survivorship care includes recovering from cancer and promoting health.

Cancer survivors

Over the past 40 years, cancer care has greatly improved. Cancer screening is finding cancer at early stages when it can be fully removed. Newer treatments are more precise and better at stopping cancer growth.

With better cancer care, people with cancer are living longer. As a result, the needs of the cancer community have changed. More people need help to recover from cancer and its treatment and to be healthy.

The term "cancer survivor" was proposed in the 1980s. The intent of the term was to raise awareness of better outcomes and changing needs. A person with cancer is a survivor:

- starting at the time of diagnosis,
- during and right after treatment, and
- through the balance of their life.

Some people do not like or identify with the term survivor. It is not meant to be a label. Its purpose is to identify the community of people with a history of cancer. Having a common term is useful for improving the care of survivors.

Survivorship care

The large and rising number of cancer survivors need survivorship care. Survivorship care improves health, wellness, and quality of life. Standards of survivorship care are listed in Guide 1.

Prevention

Prevention of a new or recurring cancer is a key part of survivorship care. You can reduce your risk of cancer with healthy living. Healthy living includes physical activity, eating well, and not using tobacco.

Less often, medical treatments are used to prevent cancer. Some people have surgery to remove a body part, like a breast, where cancer is likely to start. Some people take medication

Guide 1 **Standards for survivorship care**
Prevention of new and recurrent cancers
Prevention of late effects of cancer and treatment
Routine testing for the return of a cancer (surveillance)
Routine testing for new cancers (screening)
Assessment and treatment of late effects of cancer and treatment
Coordinated care between providers
Planning for ongoing survivorship care

that lowers hormone levels to reduce the chance of getting cancer.

Besides cancer, other unwanted effects of treatment and cancer can occur after treatment. A goal of survivorship care is to lower your chance of having these late effects. If detected early, treatment for a late effect may reduce its impact on your life.

Cancer surveillance

Cancer that was thought to be cured can reappear on tests. The return of cancer is called a recurrence or relapse. Survivorship care includes routine checking for a recurrence. This is called surveillance. Surveillance often includes updating your health history and a physical exam. Some survivors get blood tests or imaging like x-rays or scans.

Screening for cancer

Cancer screening is routine testing of cancer or pre-cancer conditions. The aim is to detect cancer at an early stage when treatment works best. There is screening for prostate, breast, cervical, skin, lung, and colorectal cancers. Screening is started when there is an average or high risk of cancer. Ask your health care provider what screening, if any, you need.

Survivors have a higher risk of a new (second) cancer. Ask your health careprovider about your chance of getting a second cancer.

- Some causes of a first cancer may be related to getting a second cancer.
- Some cancer treatments may increase cancer risk. Such treatments include radiation therapy, certain chemotherapies, and certain targeted therapies.
- Excess radiation from a lifetime of computed tomography (CT) scans slightly increases cancer risk. Ask your provider if these scans are needed and for how long.

Some survivors are at risk of hereditary cancers. Hereditary cancer is caused by abnormal genes that are passed down from parents to children. Cancers that can be hereditary include breast, ovarian, colorectal, and prostate cancer.

At health visits, update your health care providers on any new cancers among your blood relatives. Your provider may suggest getting genetic testing. A blood sample is needed. You may talk with a genetic counselor to discuss your family's cancer history.

Late effects

Many effects of treatment quickly resolve after treatment ends. An example is nausea and vomiting. Long-term effects start during treatment and persist after treatment is done. Less often, effects start long after treatment has ended. During health visits, your health care providers will assess for such late effects. They will provide treatment for late or long-term effects as needed.

Coordinated care

Cancer survivors often receive care from multiple providers. You may receive care from oncologists, a primary care provider, and non-cancer specialists. Your providers will work together and clarify their roles to address all your needs. Over time, your primary care provider will resume charge over your health care. You'll see your cancer doctor less often or if new symptoms arise.

Ongoing planning of care

A key part of survivorship care is ongoing planning of your health care. Your cancer or primary care provider will assess your needs. See one or both of them at least once a year. They will review your cancer care, health history, current abilities, and medications.

Your provider will review the plan with you. You will be given a schedule of follow-up visits, such as cancer surveillance and screening. Possible late effects may be included in the plan. Your providers may refer you to other specialists and community resources.

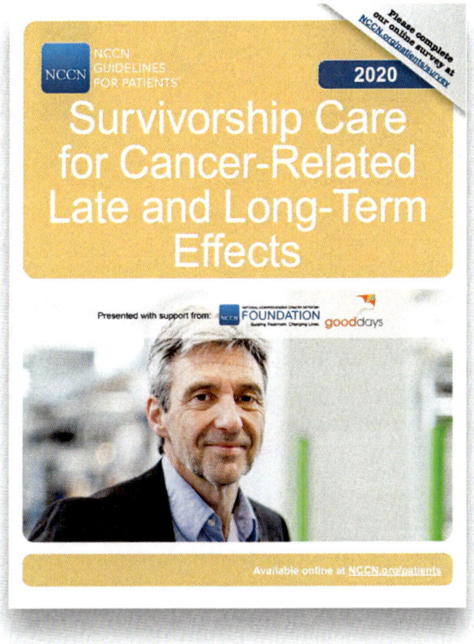

Survivorship guidelines

There have been challenges to putting survivorship care into practice. One of the strategies to overcome these challenges is practice guidelines.

Practice guidelines include recommendations by experts of the best options for care. They are based on health research, such as clinical trials. Providers use practice guidelines to tailor health care to each person.

NCCN has practice guidelines on survivorship for health care providers. The guidelines:

- Pertain to survivors with an onset of cancer in adulthood
- Apply whether treatment is ongoing, paused, stopped, or completed
- Address general survivorship issues, late and long-term effects, and healthy living
- Include screening, testing, and treatment options
- Complement treatment guidelines for cancer

NCCN has a two-part book series for survivors that are based on the practice guidelines. This survivorship book focuses on healthy living. Read about common effects in *NCCN Guidelines for Patients: Survivorship Care for Cancer-Related Late and Long-Term Effects*, available at NCCN.org/patientguidelines.

Healthy living

Cancer survivors can improve their health and quality of life with healthy living. For some cancers, healthy living lowers their risk of recurrence and death. NCCN encourages all survivors to adopt a healthy lifestyle.

There are many parts to healthy living. In the next chapters, there is detailed information on physical activity, food, supplements, weight, and metabolism. A list of basic goals for healthy living is in Guide 2.

Healthy living can be hard to do. Your care providers can be supportive. They may work with you so you can make changes on your own. At times, they may refer you to a counselor. Through counseling, you can learn about barriers to achieving goals and how to overcome them.

Guide 2 Goals of healthy living
Be physically active and avoid inactivity
Eat healthful foods
Limit or avoid drinking alcohol
Achieve and maintain a normal body weight
Don't smoke, chew, or sniff tobacco
Practice sun safety by using sunscreen and do not use tanning beds
Get enough sleep
See your primary care provider on a regular basis
Follow health guidelines as appropriate

Review

- A person with cancer is a survivor starting at diagnosis and through the balance of their life.
- Survivorship care is needed for the large and rising number of survivors. It improves health, wellness, and quality of life.
- Prevention of new and recurrent cancers is part of survivorship care. One way to lower your chance of cancer is through healthy living.
- Survivorship care includes routine testing, called surveillance, for a recurrence.
- Survivors are at higher risk for a second cancer. Follow cancer screening recommendations. If needed, genetic testing can confirm if you are at risk for hereditary cancer.
- Your health care providers will assess for late effects of cancer and its treatment. They will prescribe care to relieve or treat late effects.
- Your team of care providers will work together to meet your needs. They will clarify their roles in your care. Over time, your primary care provider will resume charge of your health care.
- Planning of survivorship care is ongoing. Survivorship plans often include follow-up visits, possible late effects, and referrals to specialists.
- There have been challenges to putting survivorship care into practice. To address these challenges, NCCN produces practice guidelines on survivorship for health care providers. The practice guidelines have been adapted into a two-part book series intended for cancer survivors.
- This NCCN book for survivors is about healthy living. Healthy living can be hard to do. Your providers can offer support including referral to a counselor.

"

DO NOT be afraid to ask your medical team ANY questions at any time!!! Your questions will help you and them. No question is stupid. Managing and or controlling your anxiety when it peaks is one thing you can control.

– Steve
Cancer survivor

2

Physical activity

13 Getting fit

14 Assessment of activity

15 Activity goals

18 Cancer-related challenges

19 Tips for achieving goals

19 Review

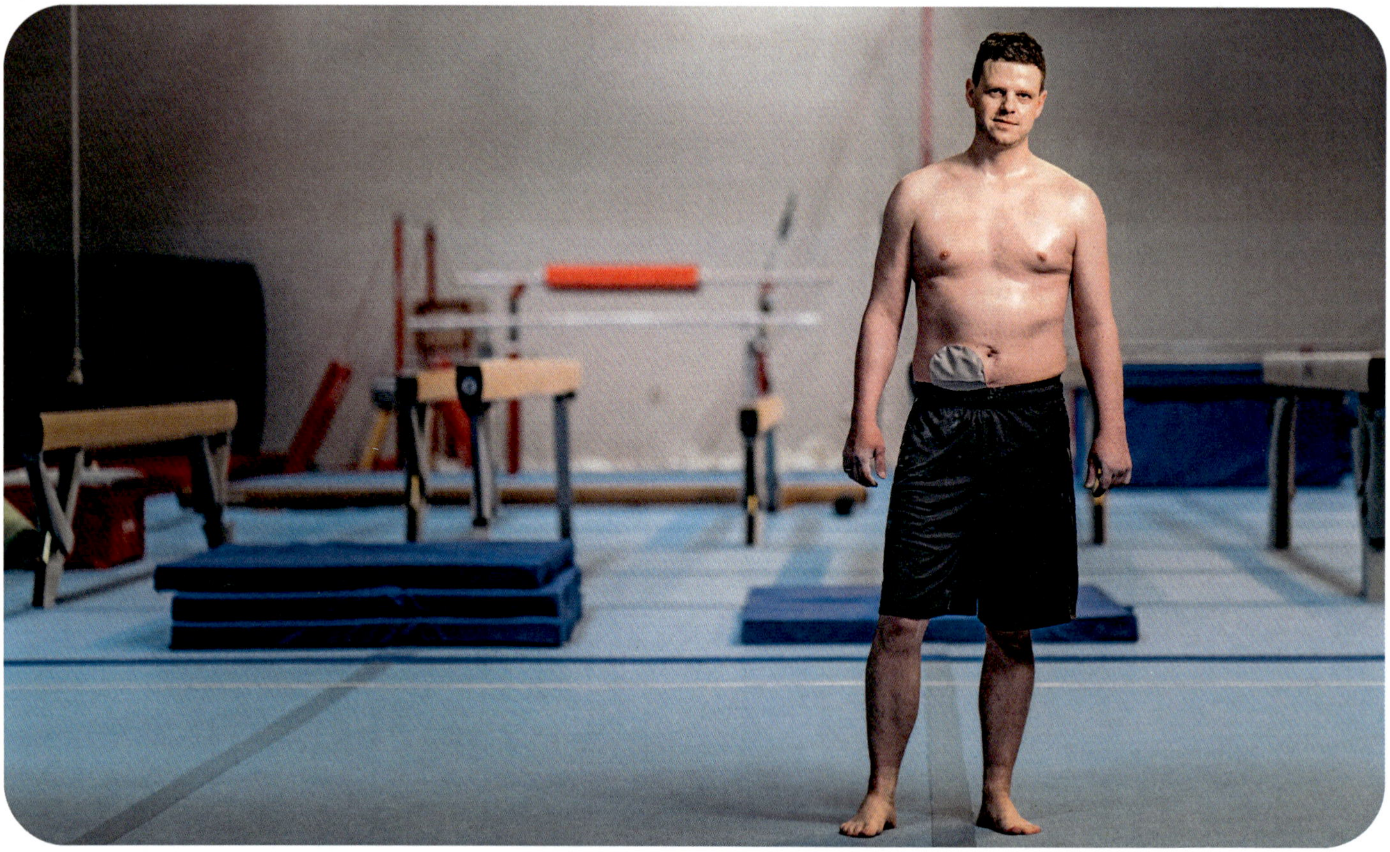

Move more! Physical activity is safe and improves the health of most cancer survivors. This chapter will help you to be more active.

Getting fit

Physical activity is any movement you make that burns more calories than when you're at rest. It includes many types of activities.

- Routine activities, such as household chores
- Recreational activities, such as swimming
- Exercise, such as brisk walking

Cancer and its treatment may limit the physical activity of cancer survivors. Reduced physical activity can result in loss of fitness and strength. With the right support, many cancer survivors can increase their physical activity. Physical activity should be a goal for most cancer survivors.

- Physical activity is safe.
- Physical activity is helpful.
- Physical activity can be achieved.

Physical activity improves the health and well-being of cancer survivors. More research is needed, but physical activity may help stop some cancers from returning in survivors and extend life. The known benefits of physical activity among survivors are listed in Guide 3.

Guide 3
Benefits of physical activity among cancer survivors

Improved cardiovascular fitness	Cardiovascular fitness is how well your body takes in and transports oxygen to tissue.
Greater muscle strength	Muscle strength is how well you can move or lift objects.
Better balance	Balance is how well you can control your body's position.
Healthier body composition	Body composition is the amount of fat, muscle, bone, and water in your body.
Less fatigue	Fatigue is being tired despite getting enough sleep.
Better emotional well-being	Emotional well-being is a balance between positive and negative feelings and being happy and satisfied with life.
Improved quality of life	Quality of life is your belief that you have a good life.
Lower risk of cardiovascular events	Cardiovascular events are medical conditions that can damage the heart.

Assessment of activity

See your cancer or primary care provider before starting new physical activity. They can provide guidance. Some people also receive support from a provider trained in exercise, such as:

- A physical therapist
- An occupational therapist
- A certified exercise professional
- A rehabilitation specialist

Exercise providers can receive training to work with cancer survivors. The American College of Sports Medicine (ACSM) and American Physical Therapy Association (APTA) offer specialty training. Search for an ACSM- or APTA-certified provider near you.

To help you plan routine physical activity, your provider may do an assessment. The assessment may include your:

- Readiness to be physically active
- Prior and current physical activity
- Barriers to physical activity
- Physical health and treatment
- Mental health and treatment

You may have barriers to getting enough physical activity. You may not have time. You may not have space in your home. You may not know what physical activities are good and safe for you.

Most cancer survivors can exercise safely. Some may need a trained professional to supervise them. Before starting physical therapy, check with your provider if you have the following.

- History of lung or major abdominal surgery
- Ostomy bag
- Cardiopulmonary disease
- Severe fatigue
- Ataxia
- Severe nutritional deficiencies
- Worsening health

> "Often times we do not want to be outside or go to the gym. A big help was online exercise videos. You can walk a mile and do a cardio exercise, just in a few minutes from your home. These were instrumental in allowing me to get my exercise from the comforts of my home—at my own pace.
>
> – Judith
> Cancer survivor

Activity goals

Your plan for physical activity should be based on your abilities and wishes. It can be tailored to how often and how intensely you want to be active. You can also help select the type of physical activity. Work with your provider to set short- and long-term goals. General goals for physical activity for cancer survivors are listed in Guide 4.

Move more, rest less often

A person can be physically active but still have long periods of inactivity. Inactivity is resting while sitting, reclining, or lying down. Prolonged inactivity on a regular basis is linked to poor outcomes. It raises the risk for new cancers and death among cancer survivors. It is linked to depressed mood and lower quality of life. General goals are to move more and not to be inactive for long periods of time.

Increase your heart rate

Any physical activity is better than none. To further improve your fitness, do activities that increase your heart rate. Among the 3 groups of physical activity, moderate and vigorous activities get the heart pumping.

- Light activity is movement that doesn't cause any change in breathing
- Moderate activity is movement during which you can talk but can't sing
- Vigorous activity is movement that makes it hard to breath when talking

A general goal is to do physical activity at a moderate or vigorous intensity during the week. At least 150 to 300 minutes of moderate-intensity activity is recommended. That's at least 2½ to 5 hours a week. If you choose vigorous-intensity activity, 75 minutes is recommended. You could also do a mix

Guide 4 General goals of physical activity for cancer survivors
Be physically active every day—routine activities, recreation, or exercise
Avoid being inactive for long periods each day
Increase your heart rate each week Option 1 Moderate-intensity activity for at least 150 to 300 minutes a week Option 2 Vigorous-intensity activity for 75 minutes a week Option 3 Mix of moderate- and vigorous-intensity activity
Strengthen major muscles with resistance training 2 to 3 times a week
Stretch major muscles on at least 2 of the days of higher-intensity activity

of moderate- and vigorous-intensity activity. Examples of physical activity are listed in Guide 5.

Strengthen and stretch your muscles

Strengthening and stretching muscles is often included in physical activity programs. Having stronger muscles may help you to do self-care activities, not fall down, and have higher bone density. Stretching increases flexibility, which is an important part of physical fitness.

All major muscle groups should be strengthened and stretched.

- Chest
- Shoulders
- Arms
- Back
- Core
- Legs

Guide 5
Examples of physical activty by intensity

Light intensity	Moderate intensity	Vigorous intensity
Slow walking	Brisk walking	Race walking
Slow biking	Biking on flat ground	Biking fast
Gentle yoga	Vinyasa yoga	High-intensity yoga
Tai chi	Pilates	Martial arts
Light housework	Light gardening	Heavy gardening
Bowling	Volleyball	Jogging, running, jumping rope
Playing catch	Baseball, softball	Running sports
Child care	Ballroom or line dancing	Fast dancing
Active gaming	Doubles tennis	Singles tennis
	Water aerobics	Fast swimming
	Using a manual wheelchair	Hiking uphill, stair climbing

Resistance training increases muscle strength. It may include using weights, elastic bands, or your own body weight to work your muscles.

- Do resistance training 2 to 3 times a week.
- Do stretching exercises on 2 of the days of higher-intensity activity.

Contact a trained provider if you're new to resistance training. You'll be given exercises to do. It is common to do 2 to 3 sets of the exercises and 10 to 15 repetitions of each exercise per set. Rest 2 to 3 minutes between sets. Resistance may be increased if the exercises become too easy.

"

I remember not being able to physically climb stairs, but today, after treatment, things are getting better and easier to navigate.

– Natalie
Cancer survivor

Strengthen muscles

Resistance training increases muscle strength. It may include using weights, elastic bands, or your own body weight to work your muscles. Do resistance training 2 to 3 times a week.

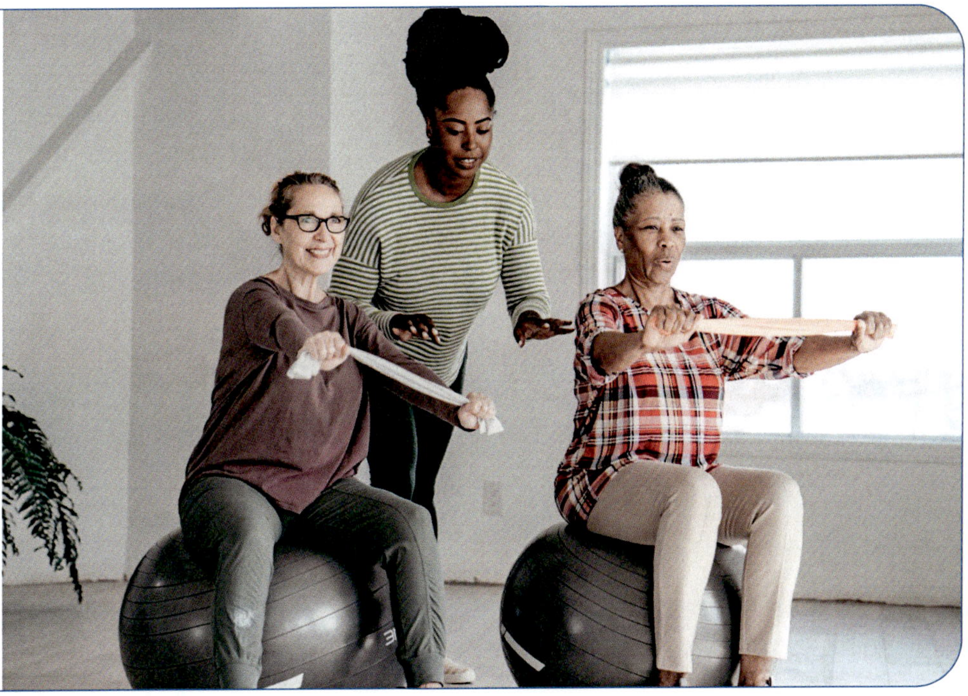

Cancer-related challenges

Cancer and its treatment can make physical activity challenging. Don't get discouraged. Talk to your care provider about ways to be active.

Lymphedema

Lymphedema is a buildup of bodily fluid called lymph. It should not stop you from being physically active. Higher-intensity activity is safe. Full use of your limbs can be maintained with resistance training and range-of-motion exercises.

- Work with a trained provider if possible.
- Get checked on a regular basis for the start or worsening of lymphedema.
- Exercise limbs with lymphedema only if the lymphedema is stable.
- Stop exercising and see a lymphedema specialist if lymphedema worsens.
- Increase your strength with resistance training in small steps.
- Compression garments may be needed during resistance training.

Ostomy

An ostomy is a surgically created change in the way stool or urine leaves the body. A stoma is a hole created in the wall of the abdomen through which stool or urine passes out. You can be active while having a stoma.

- Empty the ostomy bag before exercising.
- Slowly increase strength with resistance training that is overseen by a trained provider.
- Perform core exercises that have been revised to reduce pressure on the abdomen.
- Don't do Valsalva maneuvers since you are at risk for hernias.
- Use an ostomy protector during contact sports or when there's risk for injury to the ostomy.
- Stay hydrated during physical activity, especially if you have an ileostomy.

Peripheral neuropathy

Peripheral neuropathy is a type of nerve damage. It can be caused by cancer or its treatment. Symptoms include numbness, pain, tingling, weakness, and dizziness.

- Get your stability, balance, and gait checked before starting exercise.
- Do balance training if it would be helpful.
- Use a stationary bike or do water exercises if walking is unsafe.
- Tell your care provider of any discomfort when using hand-held weights.
- Use weights with a soft covering or padded gloves if helpful.
- Use resistance training machines if they are better than other resistance methods.

Tips for achieving goals

Physical activity is a life-long pursuit. It takes effort and support to reach and maintain goals. There are many strategies you can use to achieve success.

- Have a plan for physical activity that is tailored to you.
- Learn what stops you from being physical active.
- Find ways to overcome barriers and get help if needed.
- Set short-term goals to achieve long-term goals.
- See a provider trained in exercise if needed.
- Give yourself credit for small and large steps toward goals.
- Follow up with your provider to assess progress.
- Find support from an exercise buddy or class.
- Use a fitness device to track activity.

Review

- There are many benefits of physical exercise for cancer survivors.
- Speak with your health care provider about physical activity before starting.
- There are exercise providers who are trained to work with cancer survivors.
- Work with your providers to make a plan for physical activity that is tailored to you.
- A plan for physical activity should include goals to move more and rest less often.
- Do physical activity that increases your heart rate every week. The goal for moderate activity, like brisk walking, is at least 150 minutes a week. Vigorous activities like running can be completed in 75 minutes.
- Strengthen and stretch all major muscles at least 2 days a week.
- Don't let cancer or its treatment stop you from being active. Talk with your care providers about ways to cope with cancer-related challenges.
- Set yourself up for success! Address barriers to physical activity. Find support. Give yourself credit for small and large steps toward goals.

3
Food and supplements

21 Know your food

23 Food groups

25 Supplement safety

25 Nutrition assessment

26 Food goals

28 Review

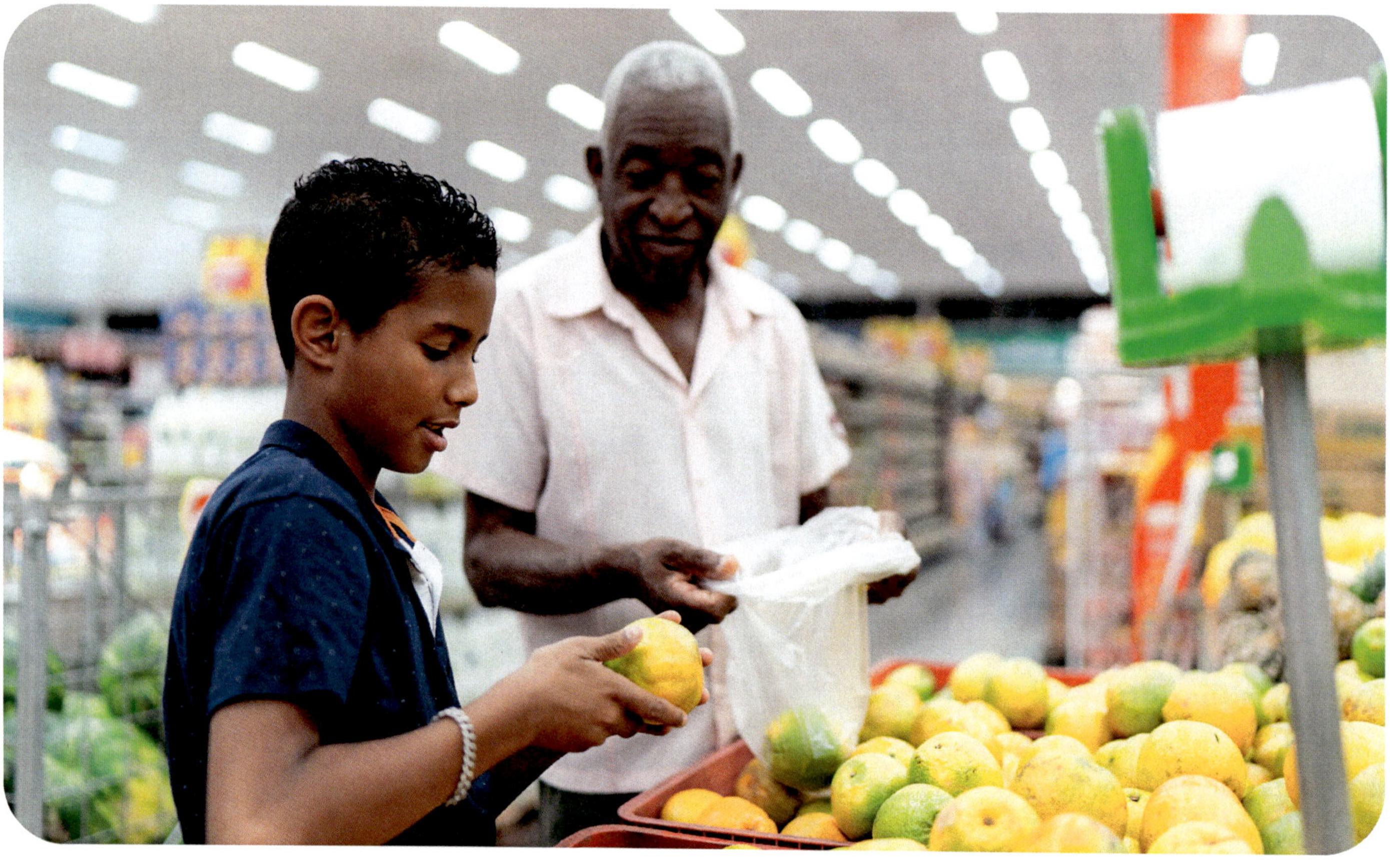

What you eat impacts your health. This chapter will help you make good food choices. It also provides guidance on supplement use.

Know your food

Eating healthful foods is key to good health. Cancer survivors are at risk for not eating the foods they need. Cancer, cancer treatments, and stress can change survivor's dietary needs and eating habits. To make good choices about food, it is important to be aware of nutrients and the food groups.

Nutrients

Nutrients are substances in food that your body uses to live. There are essential nutrients that your body can't make, so you need get them by eating food. Apart from water, there are 5 main essential nutrients.

- Fats
- Carbohydrates
- Proteins
- Vitamins
- Minerals

Essential nutrients are divided into two major classes called macronutrients and micronutrients. Macronutrients are fats, carbohydrates, and proteins. Micronutrients are vitamins and minerals.

There are more than 16 micronutrients. People only need small amounts of micronutrients, but some people still don't get enough. They are not eating foods with the micronutrients they need.

Nutrition Facts

A Nutrition Facts label is required on many packaged foods. The amount of calories and nutrients per serving are listed. Nutrition Facts can be helpful with choosing healthful foods.

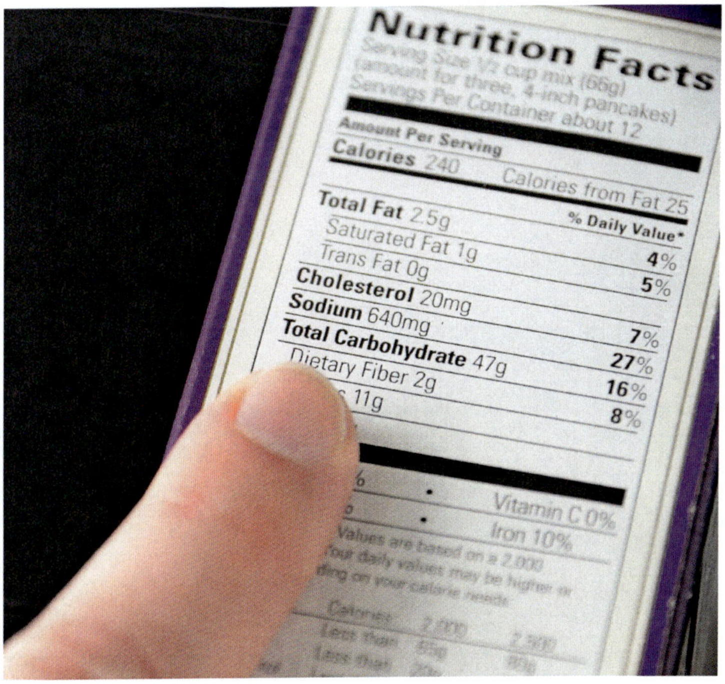

Macronutrients are needed in larger amounts because they provide energy for the body. Most people get enough or too many macronutrients in their diet. More information about macronutrients is listed in Guide 6.

Nutrition Facts labels

Nutrients are listed on the Nutrition Facts label of packaged foods. Calories are also listed. Both are listed for only a single serving. Many packaged foods have more than one serving. Take note of how many servings are in a package.

The "% daily value" tells if a nutrient is high or low per serving. A daily value of 5% or less is low. A daily value of 20% or more is high.

Guide 6
Macronutrients and healthful foods

Fats	Your body needs fats to: • grow cells, • make hormones, • absorb vitamins, • provide energy, and • keep warm.	There are 4 types: • monounsaturated fat, • polyunsaturated fat, • saturated fat, and • trans fat. Unsaturated fats are good for your health.	Foods with good fats are: • avocados, • canola oil, • fatty fish like salmon, • olive oil, and • seeds and nuts.
Carbohydrates	Carbohydrates are the main source of energy for your body.	There are 3 main types: • fiber, • starches, and • sugar. Fiber and unrefined starches are good for your health.	Foods with good carbohydrates are: • fruits, • beans and peas, • vegetables, and • whole grains.
Proteins	Your body needs proteins to: • build and repair body tissue, • fight infection, and • provide energy.	There are 9 essential proteins that you can only get from food. Foods with proteins that are low in bad fats and salt (sodium) are good for your health.	Healthful foods with proteins are: • fish, • beans and peas, • low-fat dairy foods, • nuts, and • poulty.

Food groups

It can be hard to keep track of the amount of nutrients you are eating. Food groups make choosing healthful foods easier. Food groups are everyday foods that people know.

- Fruits
- Vegetables
- Grains
- Protein foods
- Dairy

Fruits

Fruits have nutrients that are too often missing in people's diets. There are thousands of types of fruit. Fruit can be fresh, canned, frozen, and dried. Fruit can be squeezed or blended to make juice. Squeezed fruit juice lacks fiber, but a drink of 100% squeezed fruit juice counts as fruit.

Vegetables

Vegetables have many nutrients. Vegetables include dark-green vegetables, starchy vegetables, red and orange vegetables, legumes (beans and peas), and other types. Vegetables can be fresh, canned, frozen, and dried. They can be squeezed or blended to make juice. Squeezed vegetable juice lacks fiber, but a drink of 100% squeezed vegetable juice counts as a vegetable.

Grains

Grains are seeds from grasses. They include wheat, rye, rice, oats, cornmeal, and barley. Food made from whole grains has all the parts of the seeds. Refined grains have had some parts of the seeds removed. Grains have multiple nutrients including healthful carbohydrates.

MyPlate food guide

MyPlate provides information about food groups, healthful foods, and healthy food amounts. It also has many tools including recipes, learning games, and an app. Learn more about healthy eating at ChooseMyPlate.gov.

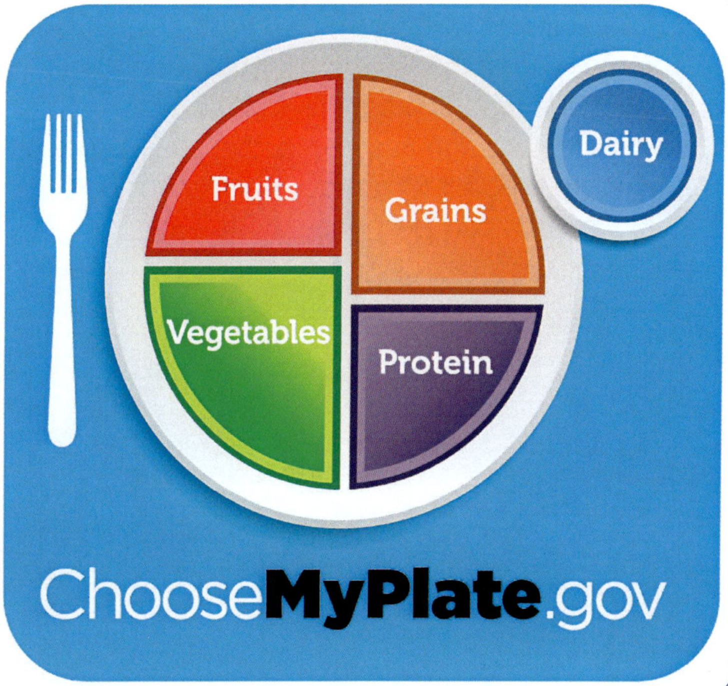

Protein foods

Proteins help almost every part of the body work. There are 9 proteins that your body can't make, so you need to eat protein foods. Foods that are nearly all protein are lean meats, poultry, fish, and egg whites. Other sources of protein are nuts, seeds, beans, peas, and soy foods like tofu.

Dairy

Dairy is a word that refers to milk and foods made from milk. Dairy provides nutrients like calcium and vitamin D. Healthful dairy choices include lower-fat milk, yogurt, and cheese. Other sources of calcium include dark leafy greens, salmon, and beans.

Food choices

In general, nutrients in each food group differ. For a healthy diet, eat a variety of food from all the food groups. When choosing food, be aware that prepared foods from stores and restaurants may have added sugar, bad fats, or high sodium.

The amount of food that is needed from each food group varies among people. It depends on factors like your age and how active you are. Learn more about food groups and making healthful food choices at ChooseMyPlate.gov.

> "Setting a goal, giving myself something positive to do, and focusing on the training for it, was very crucial for my recovery.
>
> – Chris
> Cancer survivor

Supplement safety

Supplements provide more nutrients than what is in the food you eat. They are taken by mouth in the form of a pill, capsule, tablet, or liquid. Supplements are not medicines. They are not intended to cure, treat, or prevent disease.

The U.S. Food and Drug Administration (FDA) does not approve supplements before they are sold. It has created good manufacturing practices for supplements. It also inspects the buildings and equipment used to make supplements.

There are several common types of supplements.

- Vitamin supplements
- Mineral supplements
- Essential fatty acid supplements
- Botanical supplements
- Performance and sports supplements
- Weight loss supplements
- Probiotics

Many adults take supplements. Multivitamins are most popular. Some supplements may be harmful to certain cancer survivors. Ask your care provider if any are harmful for you.

Nutrition assessment

Many cancer survivors want to have a healthier diet. You can get help from your cancer or primary care provider. Some people receive help from a registered dietician.

Registered dieticians can receive training to work with cancer survivors. They can obtain board certification as a Specialist in Oncology Nutrition. They can also become members of the Oncology Nutrition Dietetic Practice Group of the Academy of Nutrition and Dietetics.

To make a nutritional plan, your provider will do an assessment. The assessment will cover many factors related to your nutritional health.

- Day-to-day food and drink choices
- How much and how often you eat and drink
- How often you eat out
- Supplement use
- Your physical and mental health
- Treatments you've received
- Effects of diseases and treatments
- Your barriers to healthful foods and drinks

Food goals

Cancer survivors who eat healthful foods are more likely to have better outcomes. These outcomes include a decrease in cancer recurrence and new cancers. Food choices that are linked to better cancer outcomes are listed in Guide 7.

Informed choices

Knowing which foods are healthful will help you make informed choices. Ask your care providers for information on healthful foods. They may have handouts and can direct you to good websites and apps. Nutrition Facts labels are also a good resource for choosing healthful foods.

Avoid "empty-calorie" foods that have many calories and few nutrients. Instead, eat foods that are rich in nutrients compared to their calories. Nutrient-rich foods will help you get the nutrients you need. It is also helpful to eat a variety of foods since no single food has every nutrient. Learn which combinations of foods have the nutrients you need.

It is easy to overeat. You can overeat even if you eat only healthful food. Track your calories to learn how many calories are in foods and to prevent overeating.

Plant-based food

Plant-based food is made from vegetables, legumes, fruits, grains, nuts, seeds, or oils. In general, a healthy diet is rich in plant sources. Aim for at least half of your diet to be plant-based food. Most of your plant-based food should be vegetables, fruits, and whole grains.

Soy foods are made from soybeans, which are also called edamame. There is no proof from large studies that soy causes poor cancer outcomes. Eating 3 or fewer servings of soy a day is safe.

Animal-based food

Animal-based food is made from meat, poultry, fish, eggs, milk, or honey. Half or less of your diet can be animal-based food. Fish and poultry are healthy choices. Eat limited amounts of red meats and avoid processed meats.

Processed food

Processed food is food that has been changed from its natural state. There are classes of processed food.

- Minimally processed foods have been slightly changed to make prepping and cooking easier.
- Processed foods have added fats, sugar, or salt.
- Ultra-processed foods have artificial colors and flavors and preservatives.

Limit eating of processed and ultra-processed food. Drinks with lots of added sugars or fats should be consumed in small amounts.

Alcohol

Cancer survivors should limit or avoid consuming alcohol. The amount of alcohol that is safe depends on a person's biology and the cancer type. Cisgender research supports 1 drink for women and 2 drinks for men. Survivors of liver, esophageal, kidney, and head and neck cancers should not drink alcohol due to a higher chance of death.

Guide 7
General goals of food choices and supplements for cancer survivors

Informed choices	• Learn what food is healthier for you • Use Nutrition Facts labels to make healthful food choices • Eat food that is rich in nutrients • Eat many types of food • Track the number of calories you eat
Plant-based food	• Plant-based food is made from vegetables, legumes, fruits, grains, nuts, seeds, or oils • Eat plant-based food for at least half of your diet • Eat lots of vegetables, fruits, and whole grains • Eat 3 or fewer servings of soy a day
Animal-based food	• Animal-based food is made from meat, poultry, fish, eggs, milk, or honey • Eat animal-based food for half or less of your diet • Eat less than 18 ounces of red meat a week
Processed food	• Processed food is food that has been changed from its natural state • Limit the amount of processed food you eat • Avoid eating processed meat • Limit the amount of refined sugar you eat
Alcohol	• Limit or abstain from alcohol
Supplements	• Supplements are products that often contain vitamins, minerals, or herbs • Do not take supplements unless your health provider prescribes them • Do not stop eating healthful foods because you take supplements

Supplements

NCCN experts advise that most cancer survivors do not take supplements. At this time, there is no clear proof that they improve cancer prevention, control, or recurrence. Also, many supplements do not have the stated active ingredient and may have unlisted ingredients.

Supplements may be helpful for survivors who are malnourished. Survivors of stomach cancer may not be able to eat food. Survivors may have a poor diet or have health issues that require supplements. Your cancer doctor, primary care provider, or a registered dietician can provide guidance on supplements. Supplements do not replace the need for a healthy diet.

Review

- Cancer survivors are at risk for not eating the foods they need.
- Nutrients are substances in food that the body uses to live. The main nutrients are fats, carbohydrates, proteins, vitamins, and minerals. Keeping track of the nutrients in food can be hard.
- A diet based on food groups can make choosing healthful foods easier. The food groups are fruits, vegetables, grains, protein foods, and dairy.
- Supplements provide more nutrients than what is in the food you eat. The FDA does not approve supplements before they are sold.
- Work with your care provider to make a plan for eating healthful foods. Registered dieticians can earn board certification to work with cancer survivors. Your provider will perform an assessment that is used to guide planning.
- Learn about healthful foods so you can choose your meals wisely. It may be helpful to track the amount of calories in food to prevent overeating.
- At least half of your diet should consist of plant-based foods. Limit or avoid eating red meat and processed foods and drinking alcohol.
- Most cancer survivors do not need supplements. Talk with your care providers about which, if any, supplements are good for you.

"

While cancer survivors may never return to their life exactly as it was before, part of their new lives, hopefully, can be the mutual support of each other and support of patients currently battling cancer.

– Taylor
Caregiver

4

Weight and metabolism

30 Weight and metabolism goals

31 Health assessment

32 Strategies that work

34 Review

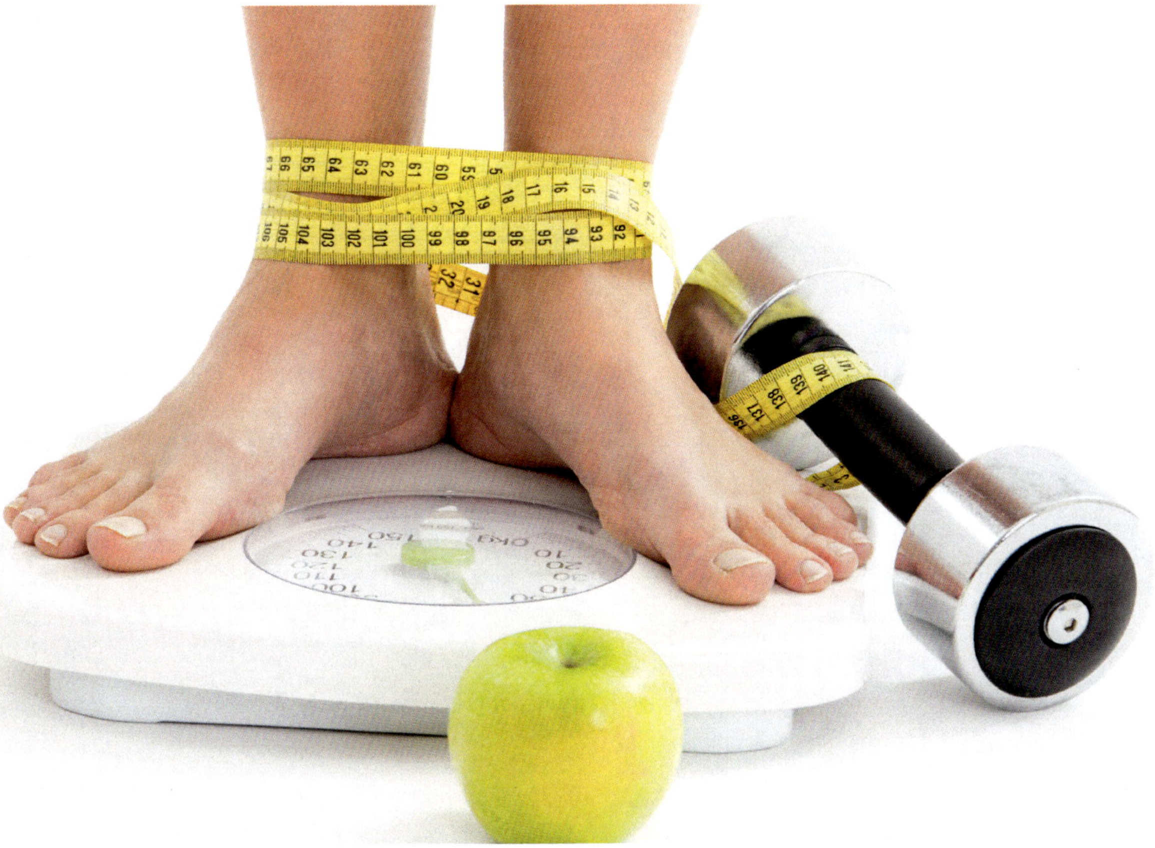

Weight is an issue for many cancer survivors. Survivors may also have poor metabolic health. This chapter explains strategies to control your weight and metabolism.

Weight and metabolism goals

Many cancer survivors experience changes in weight. Some survivors lose weight. Other survivors gain weight. Weight change may worsen a survivor's health and quality of life. It may impact cancer recurrence and survival. To improve outcomes, there are 3 goals for cancer survivors.

- Achieve a normal weight
- Maintain a normal weight
- Strive for metabolic health

BMI

Body mass index (BMI) is a quick measure of body fat based on height and weight. It is used to identify weight status.

- A BMI of 30 or more is obese
- A BMI of 25 to 29.9 is overweight
- A BMI of 18.5 to 24.9 is normal weight
- A BMI of less than 18.5 is underweight

BMI is a helpful but imperfect measure. It may be too imprecise for people who are muscular. Measuring the size of the waistline may be better. Cisgender research supports that a waist bigger than 35 inches for women and 40 inches for men increases risk for disease.

Metabolic health

Metabolism is the chemical processes in the body that are needed to live. A healthy

BMI formula

BMI is based on weight and height. In the metric formula, weight is measured in kilograms and height in meters. It can also be calculated by weight in pounds and height in inches if multiplied by 703. Learn your BMI with the online calculator at cdc.gov/healthyweight/assessing/bmi/adult_bmi/english_bmi_calculator/bmi_calculator.html.

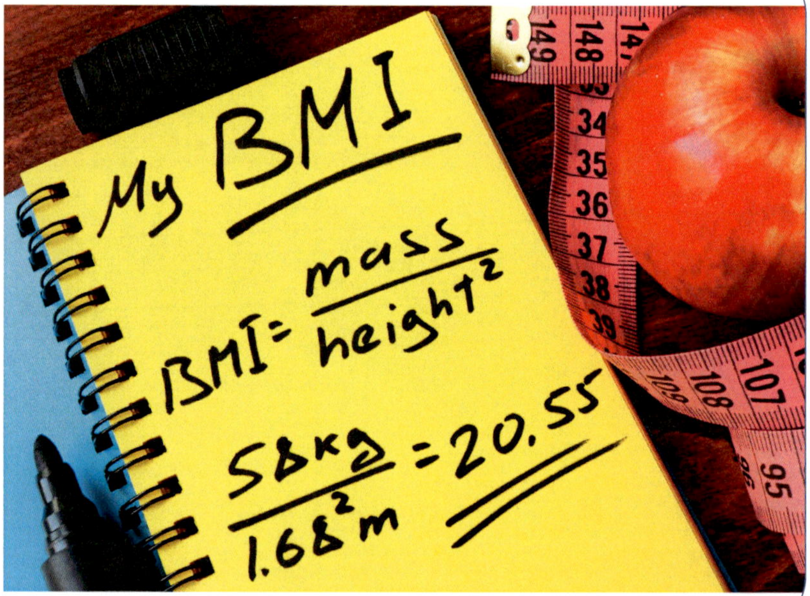

metabolism lowers the chance of heart disease, diabetes type 2, and stroke.

Metabolic syndrome is a state of unhealthy metabolism. It is diagnosed when a person has at least 3 out of 5 unhealthy metabolic conditions.

- A large waistline
- High blood pressure (hypertension)
- High blood sugar (hyperglycemia)
- High blood fats called triglycerides
- Low "good" cholesterol called HDL

You can improve your metabolic health with a healthy lifestyle. Being at a normal weight is a key goal but not the only one. Some people at a normal weight have metabolic disease. It is also important to be active, eat well, and not smoke.

Health assessment

Cancer and primary care providers can help you with weight and metabolic health. They may refer you to a specialist like a registered dietician. Look for a dietician who is board certified as a Specialist in Oncology Nutrition or a member of the Oncology Nutrition Dietetic Practice Group of the Academy of Nutrition and Dietetics.

Together, your care providers will track your BMI and metabolic health. They will also track your body composition. Body composition is often divided into fat and fat-free mass.

If your test results are of concern, your provider will perform an in-depth assessment. The assessment will be used to make a plan to improve results. The assessment will cover many factors.

- Food choices and eating habits
- Supplement use
- Levels of physical activity
- Prior weight issues and management
- Barriers to healthful eating and activity
- Readiness to change
- Physical health and treatment
- Mental health and treatment
- Dental health

"

Think of cancer as a springboard to the root cause of your underlying health condition and the healing process becomes an invitation for you to understand and improve your life on every conceivable level.

– Joe
Cancer survivor

Strategies that work

There are many strategies of weight management. They differ based on whether the goal is to gain, maintain, or lose weight. See Guide 8 for a list of key strategies.

Strategies for all survivors

Being physically active and eating healthful foods are key for all cancer survivors. Follow the goals for physical activity and healthful foods listed in **chapter 2** and **chapter 3**.

- Move more, rest less
- Exercise weekly
- Stretch and strengthen muscles
- Eat plant-based food for at least half of your diet
- Limit eating of soy, red meat, and processed meat

Guide 8
Strategies for weight management

Strategies for all survivors	• Follow the goals of physical activity listed in **chapter 2** • Follow the goals of food choices listed in **chapter 3** • Track weight, diet, calories, and physical activity
Strategies to gain weight	• Eat more often • Eat food that is high in calories and nutrients • Don't drink while eating • Address physical, mental, and social reasons of being underweight • See a registered dietician
Strategies to lose weight	• Check your weight every day • Lose no more than 2 pounds a week if younger than 65 years of age; lose no more than 1 pound a week if 65 years of age or older • Don't eat too many high-calorie foods, especially empty-calorie foods • Control how much you eat by following plate or serving size standards • Address physical, mental, and social reasons of being overweight • See a registered dietician or join a weight management program • Use community resources • Undergo bariatric surgery or take weight-loss medications if needed • Don't use weight loss supplements
Strategies to maintain weight	• Make maintaining normal body weight a goal • Check your weight every week • Don't eat too many high-calorie foods, especially empty-calorie foods • Control how much you eat by following plate or serving size standards

Another helpful strategy is to track your weight, calories, and physical activity. There are many good tracking apps. If an app is not for you, ask your provider for a handout.

Strategies to gain weight

To gain weight, you need to consume more calories. Eat more often and eat foods high in calories and nutrients. Also, don't drink while eating. Drinking may limit how much you eat. Get the help you need. Registered dieticians can provide information, guidance, and support.

Strategies to lose weight

Stay focused and weigh yourself every day. Don't feel bad if your weight is higher on one day. Instead, look for trends in weight change. Slower weight loss is healthier than fast weight loss.

To lose weight, you need to consume fewer calories. Avoid high-calorie foods and don't eat too much. Following standard serving sizes and using portion-control plates may be helpful.

Get the help and support you need. Registered dieticians help many people lose weight. Weight management programs are also popular. For some people, surgery or medications may help to lose weight. Weight loss supplements are not recommended as there is no proof that they help cancer survivors.

Strategies to maintain weight

It is important to make maintaining a normal weight a lifetime goal. Weigh yourself every week. Otherwise, you may be unaware of losing or gaining weight. To maintain weight, be careful not to eat too many foods that are high in calories. Also, be careful not to overeat or deprive yourself of food. Following serving size standards and using portion-control plates may be helpful.

Food and activity app

An app can make tracking your health goals much easier. It can count steps, scan bar codes on food, and count calories. Check out a food and activity app for cancer survivors at livestrong.com/myplate.

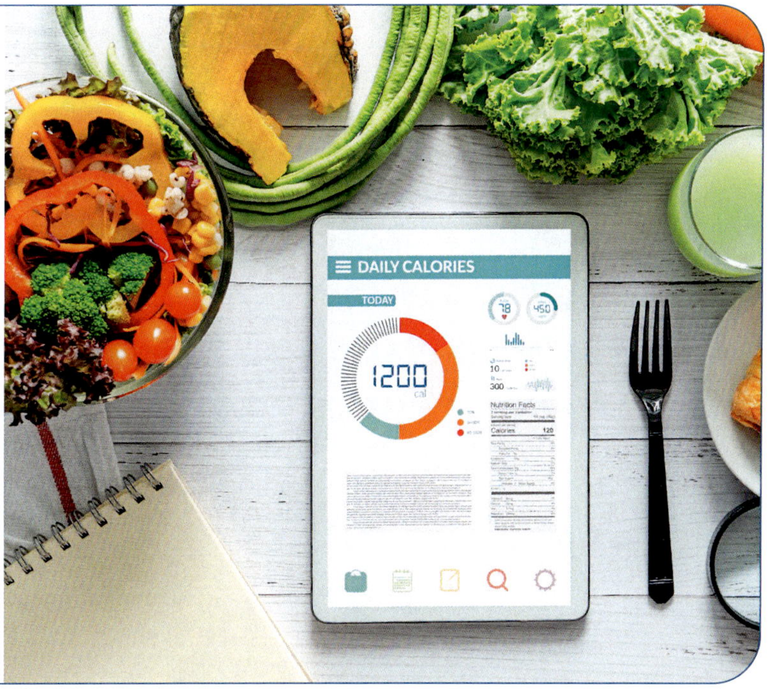

Review

- Many cancer survivors lose or gain too much weight. Being underweight or overweight is linked to poor health.
- BMI is a measure of body fat. It is based on a person's weight and height. A BMI of 18.5 to 24.9 is considered normal weight. Normal weight is a goal of healthy living for cancer survivors.
- Metabolism is the chemical processes in your body that are needed to live. Striving for metabolic health is a goal of healthy living for cancer survivors.
- Your care providers will track your BMI, metabolic health, and body composition.
- Metabolic health can be improved with a healthy lifestyle. Maintaining a normal weight is a key goal. It is also important to be active, eat healthfully, and not smoke.
- To manage weight, be active and eat healthful foods. For help meeting goals, track your weight, diet, calories, and activity levels.
- Strategies to gain weight include eating more often, eating high-calorie, healthful foods, and not drinking while eating.
- Strategies to lose weight include not eating high-calorie foods and limiting portions. Check your weight every day and don't lose weight too quickly.
- Strategies to maintain weight include checking your weight weekly, avoiding high-calorie foods, and controlling food portions.

"

Find joy by giving joy. It helps redirect your focus from what you may not be able to control to what you can.

– Sonia
Cancer survivor

5 Preventing infections

36 Immune response
37 Protect yourself
39 Safe vaccines
40 Review

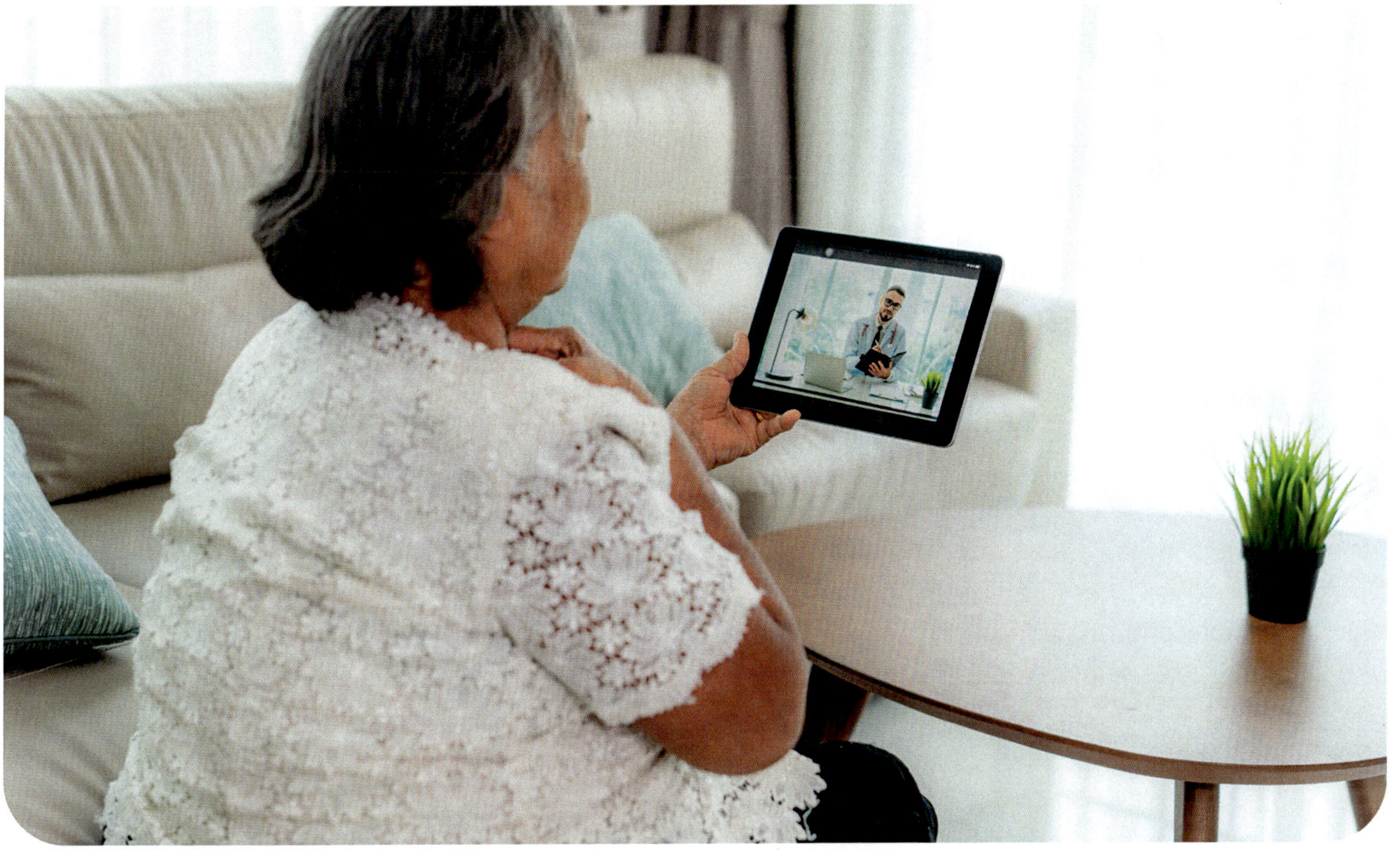

Infections can cause serious health problems. This chapter tells you how to prevent getting infections. It also explains which type of vaccines to get and when.

Immune response

An infection is defined by three key features:

- A germ (microbe) enters your body
- The germ multiplies inside your body
- The germ worsens your health

An example of an infection in people is chicken pox. Chicken pox is caused by a virus, called the varicella-zoster virus. When the virus has multiplied, it causes an itchy skin rash and flu-like symptoms. It may reactivate later in life as shingles.

The immune system is the body's defense against infections. It tries to keep germs out of your body and attacks germs that get in. Immune cells damage and kill germs. Signs that your body is fighting an infection include fever, sneezing, coughing, inflammation, and thick, yellow mucus.

Cancer survivors may be at risk for infection and a poor immune response. Immune responses can be weak during several types of cancer treatment. The time for the immune system to recover after treatment varies between treatments. Read Guide 9 for a list of cancer-related factors that can weaken the immune system.

Guide 9 Cancer-related immune suppressors
Blood cancers and cancers that spread to bone
Splenectomy
Radiation therapy
Certain chemotherapies
Certain antibody therapies
Corticosteroids, "steroids" for short
Blood stem (hematopoietic) cell transplant
CAR T-cell therapy
Blood transplant

"

Being diagnosed with cancer is scary, especially during COVID-19. Having a great medical team treating me and never losing faith, has helped me during the journey to believe that I will conquer this.

– Judith
Cancer survivor

Protect yourself

Your cancer or primary care provider will assess your risk of infection and a poor immune response. Your risk depends on

- your health history,
- the type of cancer treatment and time since treatment ended, and
- exposure to germs.

Based on the assessment, your provider will present a plan to prevent infections. Ways to prevent infections are listed in Guide 10.

Avoid getting infected

One strategy is to avoid having contact with germs. Don't go to busy indoor places or use crowded transportation. Avoid travel to high-risk areas. Don't touch animal feces or fluids, which can transmit disease. Drink bottled water and don't use ice if the drinking water is unsafe.

Another strategy is to use protective gear. Wear gloves to prevent skin cuts, which increases risk of infection. Wear shoes outdoors. Wear facial masks to reduce infections of cells called spores. Wear a cap when swimming in unsafe water.

Guide 10
Preventing infections among cancer survivors

Animal care	• Wash your hands after handling animal feces • Avoid animal feces and fluids if you have a weak immune system
Travel	• Get vaccinated before traveling to high-risk areas • Take medicines that prevent infections before traveling to high-risk areas • Learn how to prevent infections from germs in water, air, and animals
Gardening	• Wear gloves to avoid cuts • Wear a mask to avoid cells called spores
Hand hygiene	• Wash your hands often to prevent getting and spreading germs • If you can't wash your hands, use hand sanitizer with at least 60% alcohol
Antimicrobial prophylaxis	• Take prescribed medicine to prevent infections
Vaccines	• Stay up-to-date with getting vaccines

If you have contact with germs, washing is very important. Wash before and after swimming. Wash your hands before and after having close contact with people and animals. If you can't wash your hands, use hand sanitizer with at least 60% alcohol.

Antimicrobial prophylaxis

Antimicrobials are drugs that kill or stunt the growth of germs. Based on your risk, your provider may prescribe an antimicrobial to prevent an infection. Antimicrobials are grouped by which type of organisms they attack.

- Antibiotics treat bacterial infections (fluoroquinolone, levofloxacin, ciprofloxacin)
- Antifungals treat fungal infections (fluconazole, posaconazole)
- Antivirals treat viral infections (neuraminidase inhibitors, acyclovir)

Vaccines

Vaccines are biological agents that prevent diseases. Many vaccines safely prevent infections in cancer survivors. Preventing infections can save lives and protect against some cancers. Unfortunately, many survivors do not get vaccinated.

Your provider will assess which vaccines you need and are safe for you. Tell your provider if you are allergic to vaccines, medications, or food. Such allergies may impact which vaccines you can receive.

Before vaccination, your immune system should be as strong as possible. Vaccines may not work well if your immune system is weak. The number of immune cells (white blood cells) in your body should be normal or stable. You must not have any ongoing infection.

5 steps to wash hands

1. **Wet your hands with clean, running water then apply soap.**
2. **Rub and lather your entire hands including back of hand, between fingers, and under nails.**
3. **Scrub for at least 20 seconds.**
4. **Rinse your hands well under clean, running water.**
5. **Dry your hands using a clean towel or air dry them.**

cdc.gov/handwashing/index.html

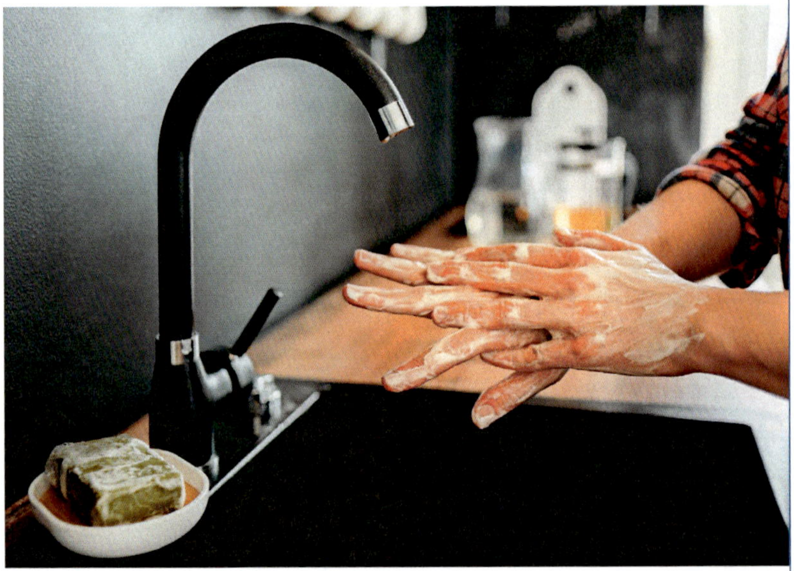

Safe vaccines

Vaccines are safe for most cancer survivors. Your provider will assess if a vaccine is safe for you based on your health. Safety also depends on the type of vaccine and time since your cancer treatment ended. Vaccines for cancer survivors are listed in Guide 11.

Types of vaccines

Vaccines prepare your body to defend against germs. They contain whole germs, parts of the germ, or a product of a germ.

There are 4 main types of vaccines.

- Live vaccines
- Inactivated vaccines
- Subunit vaccines
- Toxoid vaccines

Live vaccines contain an entire germ that has been weakened (attenuated). They create a strong immune response to the real germ. Live vaccines may cause major health problems in people with weak immune systems. Do not get live vaccines unless approved by a vaccine or cancer expert.

Guide 11
Vaccines for cancer survivors

Non-live vaccines for all survivors	• Flu vaccine every year (inactivated or recombinant) • Tdap vaccine • Recombinant zoster vaccine if you are 50 years of age or older • HPV vaccine if not received before and you are 45 years of age or younger
Non-live vaccines for survivors at high risk of certain infections	• Pneumococcal vaccine • Hepatitis B vaccine • Hepatitis A vaccine • Haemophilus influenzae type b vaccine • Meningococcal vaccine • Typhoid bacterial capsular polysaccharide vaccine • Inactivated polio vaccine • Japanese encephalitis vaccine • Rabies virus vaccine
Live vaccines to avoid or take with caution if immune system is weakened	• MMR (measles, mumps, rubella) • Oral typhoid • Rotavirus • Yellow fever • Varicella zoster

If you have a weak immune system, people who have close contact with you should not get live vaccines. If they do, keep your distance for 2 to 6 weeks depending on the vaccine. Avoid contact with feces and urine of children for 4 weeks after they get a rotavirus vaccine.

Non-live vaccines are safe for cancer survivors. Inactivated vaccines contain a germ that has been killed. Subunit vaccines contain a part of a germ. Subtypes include recombinant, polysaccharide, and conjugate vaccines. Toxoid vaccines contain a disease-causing protein from the germ. They cause a strong immune response if you are exposed to the real germ.

Timing of vaccinations

The immune system is weak during some cancer treatments. It may remain weak for a time after treatment ends. Vaccines are less safe when your immune system is weakened. If you need a vaccine, get it when your immune system is as close to normal as possible.

Get non-live vaccines:

- At least 2 weeks before cancer treatment

  or

- At least 3 months after chemotherapy or radiation therapy when possible
- At least 6 months after a blood stem cell transplant
- At least 6 months after chemotherapy and the last dose of anti–B-cell antibody therapy

If needed, you may be able to receive some vaccines during cancer treatment. An example is an inactivated flu shot. If you had a blood stem cell transplant, a flu shot should be delayed until at least 4 months after the transplant.

Get live vaccines:

- At least 4 weeks before treatment or
- At least 3 months after chemotherapy

Do not get live viral vaccines after a transplant if you have active graft-versus-host disease (GVHD) or a weakened immune system. Talk to your transplant specialist about which vaccines are safe.

Review

- The immune system is your body's natural defense against infections.
- Cancer survivors may be at risk of infections and poor immune responses.
- You can protect yourself by avoiding contact with germs, washing your hands, and taking medicines that prevent infections.
- When possible, get vaccines that do not contain a live germ. Consult with an expert in vaccines or cancer before taking live vaccines. Close contacts should also not get live vaccines.
- Do not get vaccines during cancer treatment if possible. It is safe to get them weeks before treatment or several months after treatment. If needed, you can get some types of vaccines during treatment.

6 Resources

42 Survivorship
43 Food
43 Physical Activity
43 Tobacco
44 Weight Management
44 Cancer-related effects
45 Support programs
45 Help lines

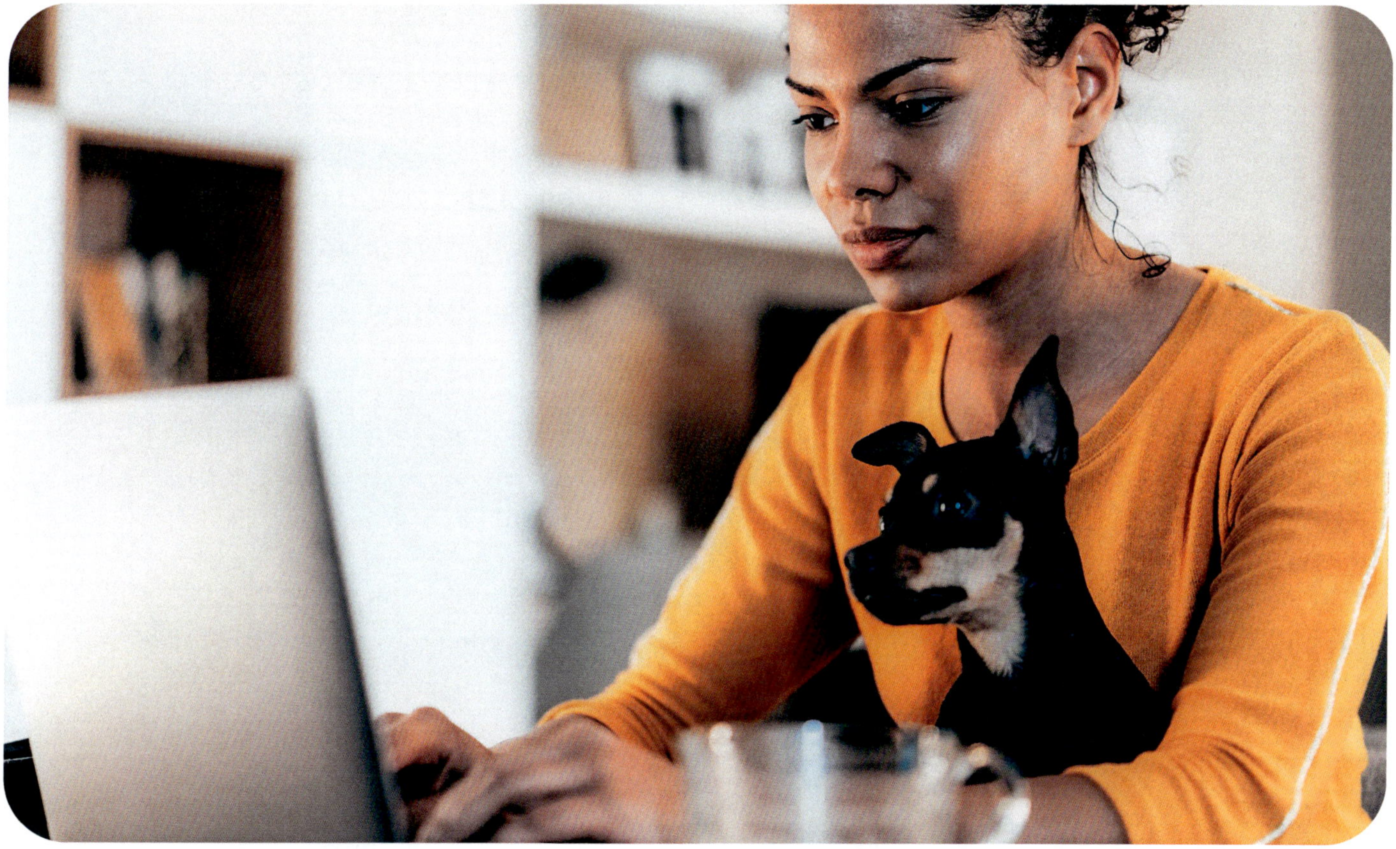

There are many resources to help you improve your health. Learn more about survivorship through the organizations listed in this chapter. Get help and use supportive tools to achieve your health goals.

Survivorship

American Institute for Cancer Research
aicr.org/cancer-survival

American Society of Clinical Oncology
cancer.net/survivorship

American Society of Clinical Oncology tracking form
cancer.net/survivorship/follow-care-after-cancer-treatment/asco-cancer-treatment-and-survivorship-care-plans

Be the Match®
bethematch.org/survivorship

Cancer Hope Network
cancerhopenetwork.org/get-support

Cancer Survivors Network
csn.cancer.org

Centers for Disease Control and Prevention
cdc.gov/cancer/survivors/index.htm

Children's Oncology Group
survivorshipguidelines.org

Leukemia & Lymphoma Society
lls.org/managing-your-cancer/follow-up-care-and-survivorship

National Cancer Institute
cancercontrol.cancer.gov/ocs/resources/survivors

National Cancer Survivorship Resource Center (The Survivorship Center)
cancer.org/SurvivorshipCenter

National Coalition for Cancer Survivorship
canceradvocacy.org

Save Your Skin
saveyourskin.ca/self-care-after-cancer

Survivor.net
survivornet.com/

"

In time you breathe a little easier, you have less scans, then less appointments and transition to survivorship. I became a survivor when I could buy long term car insurance as opposed to six months at a time.

– Kathy
Cancer survivor

Food

American Cancer Society, Calorie Counter
cancer.org/healthy/eat-healthy-get-active/take-control-your-weight/calorie-counter-calculator.html

American Institute for Cancer Research
aicr.org/cancer-prevention/healthy-eating/new-american-plate

Cancer Nutrition Consortium
cancernutrition.org

Livestrong, MyPlate Calorie Tracker
cancernutrition.org

Memorial Sloan Kettering Cancer Center
mskcc.org/cancer-care/diagnosis-treatment/symptom-management/integrative-medicine/herbs/about-herbs

MyPlate app
choosemyplate.gov/startsimpleapp

Oncology Nutrition
oncologynutrition.org/erfc

Physical Activity

American Cancer Society
cancer.org/treatment/survivorshipduringandaftertreatment/stayingactive/physical-activity-and-the-cancer-patient

American Cancer Society, Exercise calculator
cancer.org/healthy/eat-healthy-get-active/get-active/exercise-counts-calculator.html

Cancer Supportive and Survivorship Care
cancersupportivecare.com/whyexercise.html

LIVESTRONG at the YMCA
livestrong.org/ymca-search

SilverSneakers
tools.silversneakers.com

Tobacco

American Cancer Society
cancer.org/healthy/stay-away-from-tobacco.html

American Lung Association
lung.org/quit-smoking

American Lung Association
freedomfromsmoking.org

American Society of Clinical Oncology
asco.org/practice-policy/cancer-care-initiatives/prevention-survivorship/tobacco-cessation-control

Livestrong MyQuit Coach
apps.apple.com/us/app/livestrong-myquit-coach-dare/id383122255

National LGBT Cancer Network
cancer-network.org/tobacco-related-cancer-project

North American Quitline Consortium
naquitline.org

Smokefree.gov
smokefree.gov

Weight Management

American Society of Clinical Oncology
cancer.net/sites/cancer.net/files/weight_after_cancer_diagnosis.pdf

CA: A Cancer Journal for Clinicians Patient Page
acsjournals.onlinelibrary.wiley.com/doi/pdf/10.3322/caac.21146

Centers for Disease Control and Prevention, Adult BMI Calculator
cdc.gov/healthyweight/assessing/bmi/adult_bmi/english_bmi_calculator/bmi_calculator.html

National Heart, Lung, and Blood Institute
nhlbi.nih.gov/health/educational/lose_wt

National Institute of Diabetes and Digestive Kidney Diseases Body Weight Planner
niddk.nih.gov/bwp

Cancer-related effects

All common effects

American Cancer Society
cancer.org/treatment/treatments-and-side-effects/physical-side-effects.html

National Cancer Institute
cancer.gov/about-cancer/treatment/side-effects

Heart and vascular effects

American Cancer Society, Heart rate calculator
cancer.org/healthy/eat-healthy-get-active/get-active/target-heart-rate-calculator.html

CardioOnc.org
cardioonc.org/patients

CardioOnc.org, Heart Risk Calculator
cvriskcalculator.com

Million Hearts
millionhearts.hhs.gov/learn-prevent/index.html

Immunotherapy effects

NCCN Guidelines for Patients: Immunotherapy Side Effects: CAR T-Cell Therapy
NCCN.org/patients/guidelines/cancers.aspx#immunotherapySECarTCell

NCCN Guidelines for Patients: Immunotherapy Side Effects: Immune Checkpoint Inhibitors
NCCN.org/patients/guidelines/cancers.aspx#immunotherapySEICI

Mental health effects

Anxiety and Depression Association of America
adaa.org/

Anxiety and Depression Association of America (ADAA) Reviewed apps
adaa.org/finding-help/mobile-apps

NCCN Guidelines for Patients: Distress During Cancer Care
NCCN.org/patients/guidelines/cancers.aspx#distress

Oral effects

National Institute of Dental and Craniofacial Research
nidcr.nih.gov/health-info/cancer-treatments/more-info

Sexual and fertility effects

Livestrong
livestrong.org/we-can-help/livestrong-fertility

OncoLink
oncolink.org/support/sexuality-fertility/sexuality

The Oncofertility Consortium
oncofertility.northwestern.edu/for-patients

Sleep effects

National Cancer Institute
cancer.gov/about-cancer/treatment/side-effects/sleep-disorders-pdq

National Heart, Lung, and Blood Institute
nhlbi.nih.gov/health-topics/education-and-awareness/sleep-health

Support programs

Cancer Hope Network Get Matched Program
cancerhopenetwork.org/get-support/get-matched

Good Days
mygooddays.org/patients

Leukemia & Lymphoma Society
lls.org/support-resources

Save Your Skin
saveyourskin.ca/patient-support-webinars

Help lines

American Cancer Society
1.800.227.2345

American Lung Association
1.800.LUNGUSA

American Psychosocial Oncology Society
1.866.276.7443

Be the Match®
1.888.999.6743

Cancer Support Community
1.888.793.9355

Leukemia & Lymphoma Society (LLS)
1.800.955.4572

Livestrong
1.855.220.7777

National Cancer Institute
1.800.4.CANCER

National Suicide Prevention Lifeline
1.800.273.TALK

Words to know

antimicrobial
A drug that kills or stunts the growth of germs.

body mass index (BMI)
A measure of body fat based on height and weight.

cancer screening
Ongoing testing to detect cancer before it causes symptoms.

cancer survivor
A person who has or had cancer.

dairy
Another name for milk and foods made from milk.

hereditary cancer
Cancer that is caused by abnormal genes passed down from parents to a child.

immune system
The body's natural defense against disease.

inactivated vaccine
A disease-preventing agent that contains a killed germ.

infection
Invasion into the body by a harmful germ.

late effect
A cancer- or treatment-related health issue that occurs long after diagnosis or treatment.

live attenuated vaccine
A disease-preventing agent that contains a weakened germ.

lymphedema
A buildup of a bodily fluid called lymph.

macronutrient
A fat, carbohydrate, or protein that your body needs to live.

metabolism
Chemical processes in the body that are needed to live.

micronutrient
A vitamin or mineral that your body needs to live.

nutrient
A substance in food that your body uses to live.

ostomy
A surgically created change in the way stool or urine leaves the body.

peripheral neuropathy
A type of nerve damage.

processed food
Food that has been changed from its natural state.

prophylaxis
Prevention of a disease.

resistance training
A set of exercises that are repeated to strengthen muscles.

saturated fat
A fat that is unhealthful when eaten in large amounts.

stoma
A surgically created hole in the wall of the abdomen.

subunit vaccine
A disease-preventing agent that contains a part of a germ.

supplement
An edible product that contain nutrients.

surveillance
Ongoing testing for the return or a worsening of cancer.

survivorship care
Interventions to improve the health and well-being of people who have or had cancer.

toxoid vaccine
A disease-preventing agent that contains a product of a germ.

trans fat
A fake fat that is bad for your health.

unsaturated fat
A type of fat that is good for your health.

vaccine
A biological agent that prevents disease.

NCCN Contributors

This patient guide is based on the NCCN Clinical Practice Guidelines in Oncology (NCCN Guidelines®) for Survivorship Version 2.2020. It was adapted, reviewed, and published with help from the following people:

Dorothy A. Shead, MS
Director, Patient Information Operations

Laura J. Hanisch, PsyD
Medical Writer/Patient Information Specialist

Erin Vidic, MA
Medical Writer

Rachael Clarke
Senior Medical Copyeditor

Tanya Fischer, MEd, MSLIS
Medical Writer

Stephanie Rovito, MPH, CHES®
Medical Writer

Kim Williams
Creative Services Manager

Susan Kidney
Graphic Design Specialist

The NCCN Guidelines® for Survivorship Version 2.2020 were developed by the following NCCN Panel Members:

*Crystal S. Denlinger, MD/Chair
Fox Chase Cancer Center

*Tara Sanft, MD/Vice-Chair
Yale Cancer Center/Smilow Cancer Hospital

Saro Armenian, DO, MPH
City of Hope National Medical Center

K. Scott Baker, MD, MS
Fred Hutchinson Cancer Research Center/ Seattle Cancer Care Alliance

Gregory Broderick, MD
Mayo Clinic Cancer Center

Wendy Demark-Wahnefried, PhD, RD
O'Neal Comprehensive Cancer Center at UAB

Kristin Dickinson, PhD, RN
Fred & Pamela Buffett Cancer Center

*Debra L. Friedman, MD, MS
Vanderbilt-Ingram Cancer Center

Mindy Goldman, MD
UCSF Helen Diller Family Comprehensive Cancer Center

Norah Lynn Henry, MD, PhD
University of Michigan Rogel Cancer Center

Christine Hill-Kayser, MD
Abramson Cancer Center at the University of Pennsylvania

*Melissa Hudson, MD
St. Jude Children's Research Hospital/The University of Tennessee Health Science Center

Nazanin Khakpour, MD
Moffitt Cancer Center

Divya Koura, MD
UC San Diego Moores Cancer Center

Allison L. McDonough, MD
Massachusetts General Hospital Cancer Center

Michelle Melisko, MD
UCSF Helen Diller Family Comprehensive Cancer Center

Kathi Mooney, RN, PhD
Huntsman Cancer Institute at the University of Utah

Halle C. F. Moore, MD
Case Comprehensive Cancer Center/ University Hospitals Seidman Cancer Center and Cleveland Clinic Taussig Cancer Institute

Natalie Moryl, MD
Memorial Sloan Kettering Cancer Center

Javid J. Moslehi, MD
Vanderbilt-Ingram Cancer Center

Tracey O'Connor, MD
Roswell Park Cancer Institute

Linda Overholser, MD, MPH
University of Colorado Cancer Center

Electra D. Paskett, PhD
The Ohio State University Comprehensive Cancer Center - James Cancer Hospital and Solove Research Institute

Chirayu Patel, MD, MPH
Massachusetts General Hospital Cancer Center

Lindsay Peterson, MD
Siteman Cancer Center at Barnes-Jewish Hospital and Washington University School of Medicine

William Pirl, MD
Dana-Farber/Brigham and Women's Cancer Center

M. Alma Rodriguez, MD
The University of Texas MD Anderson Cancer Center

Kathryn J. Ruddy, MD, MPH
Mayo Clinic Cancer Center

Lillie Shockney, RN, MAS
The Sidney Kimmel Comprehensive Cancer Center at Johns Hopkins

Sophia Smith, PhD, MSW
Duke Cancer Institute

Karen L. Syrjala, PhD
Fred Hutchinson Cancer Research Center/ Seattle Cancer Care Alliance

Amye Tevaarwerk, MD
University of Wisconsin Carbone Cancer Center

Phyllis Zee, MD, PhD
Robert H. Lurie Comprehensive Cancer Center of Northwestern University

NCCN Staff

Deborah Freedman-Cass, PhD
Manager, Licensed Clinical Content

Nicole McMillian, MS
Guidelines Coordinator

* Reviewed this patient guide. For disclosures, visit NCCN.org/about/disclosure.aspx.

NCCN Cancer Centers

Abramson Cancer Center
at the University of Pennsylvania
Philadelphia, Pennsylvania
800.789.7366 • pennmedicine.org/cancer

Fred & Pamela Buffett Cancer Center
Omaha, Nebraska
402.559.5600 • unmc.edu/cancercenter

Case Comprehensive Cancer Center/
University Hospitals Seidman Cancer
Center and Cleveland Clinic Taussig
Cancer Institute
Cleveland, Ohio
800.641.2422 • UH Seidman Cancer Center
uhhospitals.org/services/cancer-services
866.223.8100 • CC Taussig Cancer Institute
my.clevelandclinic.org/departments/cancer
216.844.8797 • Case CCC
case.edu/cancer

City of Hope National Medical Center
Los Angeles, California
800.826.4673 • cityofhope.org

Dana-Farber/Brigham and
Women's Cancer Center |
Massachusetts General Hospital
Cancer Center
Boston, Massachusetts
617.732.5500
youhaveus.org
617.726.5130
massgeneral.org/cancer-center

Duke Cancer Institute
Durham, North Carolina
888.275.3853 • dukecancerinstitute.org

Fox Chase Cancer Center
Philadelphia, Pennsylvania
888.369.2427 • foxchase.org

Huntsman Cancer Institute
at the University of Utah
Salt Lake City, Utah
800.824.2073
huntsmancancer.org

Fred Hutchinson Cancer
Research Center/Seattle
Cancer Care Alliance
Seattle, Washington
206.606.7222 • seattlecca.org
206.667.5000 • fredhutch.org

The Sidney Kimmel Comprehensive
Cancer Center at Johns Hopkins
Baltimore, Maryland
410.955.8964
www.hopkinskimmelcancercenter.org

Robert H. Lurie Comprehensive
Cancer Center of Northwestern
University
Chicago, Illinois
866.587.4322 • cancer.northwestern.edu

Mayo Clinic Cancer Center
Phoenix/Scottsdale, Arizona
Jacksonville, Florida
Rochester, Minnesota
480.301.8000 • Arizona
904.953.0853 • Florida
507.538.3270 • Minnesota
mayoclinic.org/cancercenter

Memorial Sloan Kettering
Cancer Center
New York, New York
800.525.2225 • mskcc.org

Moffitt Cancer Center
Tampa, Florida
888.663.3488 • moffitt.org

The Ohio State University
Comprehensive Cancer Center -
James Cancer Hospital and
Solove Research Institute
Columbus, Ohio
800.293.5066 • cancer.osu.edu

O'Neal Comprehensive
Cancer Center at UAB
Birmingham, Alabama
800.822.0933 • uab.edu/onealcancercenter

Roswell Park Comprehensive
Cancer Center
Buffalo, New York
877.275.7724 • roswellpark.org

Siteman Cancer Center at Barnes-
Jewish Hospital and Washington
University School of Medicine
St. Louis, Missouri
800.600.3606 • siteman.wustl.edu

St. Jude Children's Research Hospital/
The University of Tennessee
Health Science Center
Memphis, Tennessee
866.278.5833 • stjude.org
901.448.5500 • uthsc.edu

Stanford Cancer Institute
Stanford, California
877.668.7535 • cancer.stanford.edu

UC San Diego Moores Cancer Center
La Jolla, California
858.822.6100• cancer.ucsd.edu

UCLA Jonsson
Comprehensive Cancer Center
Los Angeles, California
310.825.5268 • cancer.ucla.edu

UCSF Helen Diller Family
Comprehensive Cancer Center
San Francisco, California
800.689.8273 • cancer.ucsf.edu

University of Colorado Cancer Center
Aurora, Colorado
720.848.0300 • coloradocancercenter.org

University of Michigan
Rogel Cancer Center
Ann Arbor, Michigan
800.865.1125 • rogelcancercenter.org

The University of Texas
MD Anderson Cancer Center
Houston, Texas
844.269.5922 • mdanderson.org

University of Wisconsin
Carbone Cancer Center
Madison, Wisconsin
608.265.1700 • uwhealth.org/cancer

UT Southwestern Simmons
Comprehensive Cancer Center
Dallas, Texas
214.648.3111 • utsouthwestern.edu/simmons

Vanderbilt-Ingram Cancer Center
Nashville, Tennessee
877.936.8422 • vicc.org

Yale Cancer Center/
Smilow Cancer Hospital
New Haven, Connecticut
855.4.SMILOW • yalecancercenter.org

Notes

Index

alcohol 10, 26–27

animal-based food 26–27

antimicrobial prophylaxis 37–38

body mass index (BMI) 30

cancer screening 8

exercise providers 14

food groups 23–24

immune system 36

late effects 8

lymphedema 18

metabolic health 30–31

moderate-intensity activity 15–16

NCCN Cancer Centers 50

NCCN Contributors 49

nutrients 21–22

nutrition fact labels 21–22

ostomy 18

peripheral neuropathy 18

plant-based food 26–27

practice guidelines 9

processed food 26–27

resistance training 17

sleep 10

stretching 16–17

sun safety 10

supplements 25, 27

surveillance 7–8

survivorship care 7–9

tobacco 10

vaccines 37–40

vigorous-intensity activity 15

washing hands 38

weight management 32–33

Made in United States
North Haven, CT
11 January 2024

47350564R00031